S0-BBI-451

 Bristol-Myers Squibb Company

 Otsuka America Pharmaceutical, Inc.

Dear Healthcare Professional:

Bristol-Myers Squibb Company and Otsuka America Pharmaceutical, Inc. are pleased to present you with *Pharmacologic Treatment of Schizophrenia*, Second Edition by Robert R. Conley, M.D. and Deanna L. Kelly, PharmD.

Abilify™ (aripiprazole) is co-marketed by Bristol-Myers Squibb Company and Otsuka America Pharmaceutical, Inc. This reference text includes product information that differs from the approved product labeling. Please refer to the approved Abilify™ (aripiprazole) prescribing information for complete details about indications, contraindications, precautions, and warnings.

Sincerely,

Bristol-Myers Squibb Company
and Otsuka America Pharmaceutical, Inc.

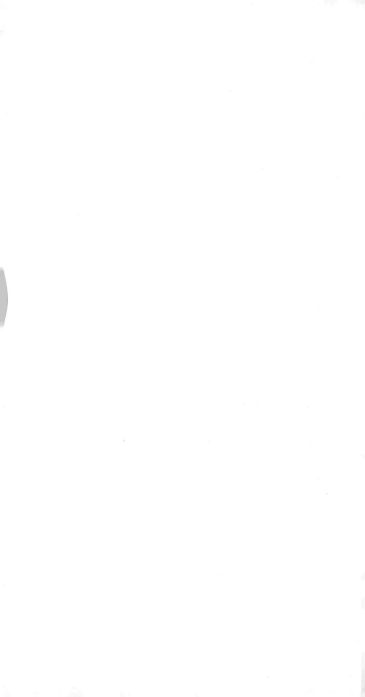

Pharmacologic Treatment of Schizophrenia

Second Edition

Robert R. Conley, MD
Director of the Treatment Research Unit
Maryland Psychiatric Research Center
Associate Professor of Psychiatry
and Pharmacy Practice
University of Maryland

Deanna L. Kelly, PharmD, BCPP
Maryland Psychiatric Research Center
Assistant Professor of Psychiatry
and Pharmacy Practice
University of Maryland

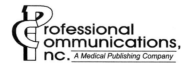
Professional
Communications,
Inc. *A Medical Publishing Company*

Copyright 2003
Robert R. Conley, MD and
Deanna L. Kelly, PharmD, BCPP

Published by
Professional Communications, Inc.

Marketing Office:	*Editorial Office:*
400 Center Bay Drive	PO Box 10
West Islip, NY 11795	Caddo, OK 74729-0010
(t) 631/661-2852	(t) 580/367-9838
(f) 631/661-2167	(f) 580/367-9989

For orders only, please call
1-800-337-9838

or visit our website at
www.pcibooks.com

ISBN: 1-884735-83-5

Printed in the United States of America

DISCLAIMER

The opinions expressed in this publication reflect those of the authors. However, the authors make no warranty regarding the contents of the publication. The protocols described herein are general and may not apply to a specific patient. Any product mentioned in this publication should be taken in accordance with the prescribing information provided by the manufacturer.

This text is printed on recycled paper.

DEDICATION

This book is dedicated to our patients and their families. We honor their struggle against the serious condition of schizophrenia.

ACKNOWLEDGMENT

We thank the National Alliance for Research on Schizophrenia and Depression (NARSAD), the Theodore and Vada Stanley Foundation, and the National Institutes of Health for their support of our work.

Much of the background for this work came from the teaching we have done in public hospitals and clinics throughout the country. We would like to thank the TRU and the staff in those sites for their questions and insight into our ideas.

Finally, we could not have completed this work without the support and encouragement of our families, and we thank them for their support. One of us (RRC) has been blessed with twin daughters, who send me away on my trips with the words, "We'll miss you, but we know your work is important, Dad." I would like to thank Anna and Sarah Conley for your words; they help more than you know.

TABLE OF CONTENTS

TABLES

viii

FIGURES

Introduction

There have been many "revolutions" in the care and treatment of people with schizophrenia over the past century. The most promising was the introduction of specific antipsychotic medications in the 1950s and 1960s. These medications, along with a marked societal change in the way the mentally ill are treated (with an emphasis on community as opposed to institutional treatment), have improved the life of most people who suffer from schizophrenia. The goal of normal functioning, however, remains elusive for most people with this illness. Unemployment, inadequate housing, and a high death rate continue to be common problems for these people. One of the major reasons for this has been that traditional antipsychotic medications, while helpful in controlling some of the obvious symptoms of schizophrenia, do not control all of the symptoms of this illness and are associated with serious lifestyle-limiting side effects.

In the 1990s and the early 2000s, a new group of antipsychotic medications were introduced, the newest of which possesses a novel mechanism of dopamine stabilization. The second-generation antipsychotic drugs are more effective and have fewer side effects than traditional medications; however, they are not a cure and may have serious side effects of their own. Furthermore, people who take these medications are generally much more capable of experiencing and showing emotions than people who take traditional medications. This helps people to live better but makes them appear much less controlled than people who take traditional medications. For this reason, clinicians must use new outcome measures to judge the effectiveness of a medication.

We hope this book helps clinicians in their search for the appropriate medication regimen for each of their patients. We need to be careful about claims that the new medications represent another revolution. We do feel, however, that most people who suffer from schizophrenia today can lead a much better life with the optimal use of the second-generation antipsychotic drugs.

This book has been prepared for clinicians as a review of the treatment and management of schizophrenia and other serious chronic psychotic disorders. The authors would like to thank the clinicians and investigators whose observations and publications have added to our own work in this exciting area. Their contributions have made this timely presentation of new pharmacotherapies for schizophrenia possible.

General Information About Schizophrenia

Epidemiology

Schizophrenia is one of the more challenging and complex psychiatric disorders that afflict humans. The core symptoms of this illness are highly variable among patients, with a wide array of symptoms such as:

- Hallucinations
- Delusions
- Disorganized speech and behavior
- Inappropriate affect
- Cognitive deficits
- Impaired psychosocial functioning.

The onset of symptoms in most cases is insidious, usually preceded by a prodromal phase characterized by:

- Gradual social withdrawal
- Diminished interests
- Changes in appearance and hygiene
- Changes in cognition
- Bizarre or odd behavior.

Descriptions of chronic severe functional psychosis date back as far as human literature. Often psychotic symptoms were considered to be signs or manifestations of supernatural influences on the individual. Psychotic individuals have held the burden of being shunned and feared by society in general. Greek physicians first wrote about the concept that mental illness was due to natural forces (eg, a disease). This concept was not embraced by Western physicians until the Renaissance but was kept alive by Arabic physicians who practiced classical medicine. During the 17th and 18th centuries, the first Western mental hospitals were established and much work went into characterizing and describing mental illness. Morel, in 1860, first proposed the term "deménce précoce" to describe a progressive insanity in the young. Kraepelin, in 1896, building on this work and that of others, such as Hecker and Kahlbaum, distinguished "dementia praecox" from manic-depressive psychosis. Kraepelin believed that this condition always progressed to marked dementia. In 1911, Eugene Bleuler coined the term schizophrenia, defining a disorder that included dementia praecox but also other forms of progressive psychosis in which the patient did not deteriorate as severely. This work gave rise to our modern concept of schizophrenia (Table 1.1). As we better understand the brain and central nervous system (CNS) pathophysiology, diagnosis and treatment will continue to change.

Pathophysiology

Advances in technology have provided a means for investigating functional and structural abnormalities in the brain through the use of:

TABLE 1.1— SUMMARY OF EPIDEMIOLOGIC FACTORS
Lifetime Prevalence   • 1% in both males and females   • Occurs in most areas of the world
Onset of Illness   • Late adolescence/early adulthood   • Earlier in males
Average Age at First Hospitalization   • Males—15 to 24 years   • Females—25 to 34 years

- Positron emission tomography (PET)
- Single photon emission computed tomography (SPECT)
- Functional magnetic resonance imaging (fMRI).

This technology has led to advancement in the field of schizophrenia research in determining areas of disturbance in certain brain regions (Table 1.2). Unfortunately, however, research in this area has not yet led to the identification of the basic neuropathology of the disorder.

TABLE 1.2 — SUMMARY OF STRUCTURAL AND FUNCTIONAL ABNORMALITIES

- Cortical atrophy (prefrontal lobe, medial temporal cortex)
- Diencephalic gliosis (hippocampus, amygdala)
- Ventricular dilation (particularly left sided)
- Cerebellar atrophy (vermis)
- Reversal of normal frontal and occipital lobe asymmetries

Functional changes in the brain of people with schizophrenia are highly correlated with certain symptoms. Therefore functional imaging has progressed along the lines of delineating the metabolic changes associated with specific symptom complexes. Positive symptoms, negative symptoms, and cognitive disturbances, all more fully described later in this chapter, are associated with specific functional changes in the brain (Table 1.3).

The introduction of effective antipsychotic medications in the mid 1950s opened the door for studies assessing neurochemical hypotheses of schizophrenia. The advent of highly sensitive assays that measure CNS neurotransmitter levels, their metabolites, and related metabolic enzymes prompted the development

TABLE 1.3 — SPECIFIC FUNCTIONAL CHANGES IN THE BRAIN		
Symptom Complex	**Brain Region**	**↑/↓ in Activity***
Thought disorder	Anterior cingulate gyrus	↑
Reality distortions/ delusions	Left prefrontal cortex	↓
Positive symptoms	Left hippocampus	↑
Auditory hallucinations	Broca's area, superior temporal cortex	↑
Negative symptoms	Left prefrontal cortex	↓
Psychomotor poverty	Inferior parietal cortex	↓
Anhedonia	Right inferior parietal cortex, cingulate gyrus	↑
* Compared with normal controls.		

of hypotheses proposing that neurotransmitters have a role in the causation of schizophrenia.

The most common pathophysiologic theories associated with the etiology of schizophrenia involve the dopaminergic system. This hypothesis began in the late 1950s when it was discovered that antipsychotic drugs are postsynaptic dopamine antagonists. It has been observed that drugs that increase dopamine will enhance or produce positive psychotic symptoms (cocaine, amphetamines) and drugs such as antipsychotics that decrease dopamine will decrease or stop positive symptoms. There are four dopamine tracts of primary interest in the brain (Figure 1.1). A basic knowledge of these tracts and their relationship is important for understanding the therapeutic and adverse effects of both traditional and second-generation antipsychotic drugs (SGADs) (Table 1.4).

FIGURE 1.1 — PRINCIPAL DOPAMINE PATHWAYS IN THE BRAIN

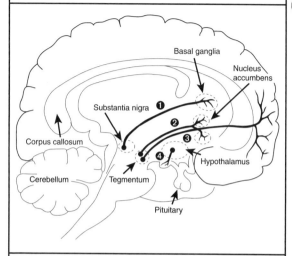

(1) The nigrostriatal tract, also known as the extrapyramidal pathway, begins in the substantia nigra and ends in the caudate nucleus and putamen of the basal ganglia. (2) The mesolimbic tract originates in the midbrain tegmentum and innervates the nucleus accumbens and adjacent limbic structures. (3) The mesocortical tract originates in the midbrain tegmentum and innervates anterior cortical areas. (4) The tuberoinfundibular tract projects from the arcuate and periventricular nuclei of the hypothalamus to the intermediate lobe of the pituitary and to the portal blood system surrounding the anterior pituitary.

Martin MB, et al. In: *Textbook of Neuropsychiatry*. Washington, DC: American Psychiatric Press; 1997:55-85.

The nigrostriatal tract originates in the A9 area of the substantia nigra and terminates with the synapses in the putamen and caudate nucleus of the basal ganglia. The mesolimbic pathway projects from the midbrain ventral tegmentum (A10) to the cingulate gyrus and limbic regions. The mesocortical tract extends

TABLE 1.4 — SUMMARY OF DOPAMINE TRACTS AND EFFECTS OF ANTIPSYCHOTICS

Dopamine Tract	Effect of Antipsychotic
Nigrostriatal	Movement disorder
Mesolimbic	Relief of psychosis
Mesocortical	Increase in negative symptoms, akathisia?
Tuberoinfundibular	Increased prolactin concentrations

from A10 to the prefrontal and frontal cortex. The tuberoinfundibular tract originates in the hypothalamus and projects to the pituitary gland.

There is much evidence supporting the dopaminergic receptor–deficit hypothesis. Increased glucose metabolism in the basal ganglia and decreased metabolism in the frontal cortex may be indicative of dopaminergic hyperactivity and hypoactivity in these regions, respectively. PET studies measuring receptor densities using dopamine $(D)_2$-specific ligands such as raclopride show increased densities of D_2 receptors in the basal ganglia and decreased densities in the prefrontal cortex. Other direct evidence supporting the validity of the dopamine hypothesis comes from postmortem evaluation of tissues and plasma. Investigators have measured the amount of dopamine and its metabolites, such as homovanillic acid (HVA). The brain of people with schizophrenia has increased presynaptic dopamine and/or HVA levels in areas of the mesocortical and mesolimbic systems as compared with that of normal controls.

The hypothesis that the dopamine system explains schizophrenia symptoms is far from complete. Recently, it has been suggested that combined dysfunction of the dopamine and glutamate transmitter systems may better explain this disorder. Phencyclidine (PCP) and ketamine are psychotomimetic drugs that noncompetitively block the ion channel of the glutamate subtype receptor, the *N*-methyl-D-aspartate (NMDA) receptor. These agents can elicit the full range of psychotic symptoms resembling those of schizophrenia. Based on this model of schizophrenia, NMDA receptor hypofunction, as a type of transmitter disturbance, may explain many of the symptoms seen in this illness. Dopamine transmission is intrinsically tied to glutamate release and may explain why medications that antagonize dopamine may partially work in this disorder. Dopamine receptors may inhibit glutamate release; thus a defect in the dopamine system that causes hyperactivity could result in excessive suppression of glutamate release at NMDA receptors. The net effect would be hypofunction of the NMDA receptor system as the basis for schizophrenic symptoms.

There has also been a great deal of speculation regarding the role of serotonin receptor antagonism in regard to antipsychotic effects. Many traditional antipsychotics are highly active at serotonin receptors, but this property does not distinguish the clinical effects of these drugs in a meaningful way. The serotonin hypothesis of psychosis actually predates the dopamine hypothesis, largely because of lysergic acid diethylamide (LSD), a drug with psychotomimetic properties that releases serotonin. Interest in this theory was rekindled by the finding that clozapine, which has a 100-fold selectivity for serotonin compared with dopamine receptors, is highly efficacious. The other SGADs also have high serotonin-to-dopamine binding ratios. Serotonin receptor binding may be important to these drugs' actions, possibly by stimulating dopamine activity in mesocortical pathways. However, a compelling theory relating dopamine and serotonin receptor affinities has not yet been developed.

Genetic Predisposition

There may be a lesion present at birth with the potential for NMDA receptor hypofunction, and this may not trigger psychopathologic or neuropathologic processes until late adolescence, at which time it would begin to trigger schizophrenic symptoms. There is fairly strong evidence that schizophrenia is at least partially genetic in nature. The risks are listed in Table 1.5.

Many genes have been weakly associated with the development of schizophrenia. However, there is probably no single "schizophrenic gene." The possible genetic effect is a susceptibility to schizophrenia, with either a certain gene or a combination of several genes necessary for development of the disorder (Table 1.6).

Clinical Presentation

Schizophrenia is a chronic disorder of thought, affect, and a significant disturbance in the individual's

TABLE 1.5 — RISKS FOR DEVELOPING SCHIZOPHRENIA	
Risk Factor	**Risk** (%)
First-degree relative is diagnosed	10
Both parents are diagnosed	40
Dizygotic twins	10
Monozygotic twins	40 to 50

TABLE 1.6 — GENES IDENTIFIED AS SCHIZOPHRENIA RELATED	
Amount of Evidence	**Genes**
Significant evidence	13, 22
Weak evidence	6, 8, 10, 14, 15

ability to function in society and develop interpersonal relationships. The clinical presentation of this disorder can be extremely varied, and despite the attempts to portray a stereotype in the media, the stereotypic schizophrenic individual does not exist. The categorization of independent pathophysiologic processes underlying signs and symptoms dates back to Kraepelin. He proposed that there were two processes characterizing schizophrenia. The first domain was a "weakening of those emotional activities which permanently form the mainsprings of volition." "Emotional dullness, loss of volition, and failure of mental activities" were the results of this domain and termed the "avolitional syndrome." This was the predecessor of the current concept of primary negative symptoms or the deficit syndrome. Kraepelin's second domain consisted of "the loss of the inner unity of the activities of intellect, emotion, and volition, in themselves and one another."

In the 1970s, Strauss and others suggested that schizophrenic symptoms fall into three specific symptom complexes: positive symptoms, negative symptoms, and disorders of relating. Carpenter and others further characterized these three symptom domains:
- Psychotic symptoms
- Cognitive symptoms
- Negative symptoms.

■ Psychotic Symptoms
The acute psychotic symptoms include:
- Hallucinations (distortion or exaggeration of perception)
- Delusions (fixed false beliefs).

Hallucinations may occur as auditory, visual, olfactory, gustatory, and tactile events, but auditory hallucinations are the most common type in patients with schizophrenia. Hearing of voices is a frequent occurrence, and they are distinct from the person's own thoughts. The content of hallucinations is variable but is often threatening or commanding. Delusions are erroneous beliefs that usually involve a misinterpretation of perceptions or experiences. Types of delusions are listed in Table 1.7.

■ Cognitive Symptoms

Subtle disturbance in associative thinking may develop years before disorganized thinking (formal thought disorder). Inferences about thought are based primarily on the individual's speech. Thinking and speech of patients are frequently incomprehensible to others and often are illogical. Characteristics of formal thought disorder are listed in Table 1.8.

■ Negative Symptoms

Primary negative symptoms or deficit symptoms are quite ubiquitous in schizophrenia; however, they are difficult to evaluate because they occur in a continuum with normality, are nonspecific, and are often due to medication side effects (secondary negative symptoms), mood disorder, environmental understimulation, or demoralization. The best test for establishing true negative symptoms is to examine their persistence for a considerable period of time despite efforts directed at resolving the other causes. Approximately 10% to 15% of schizophrenics may exhibit the majority of psychopathology as negative symptoms. Such patients may be referred to as having a "deficit syndrome" (Table 1.9).

■ Presentation of Symptoms

Patients with schizophrenia may be uncooperative, hostile, and verbally or physically aggressive due to their misinterpretation of reality and often due to command hallucinations. Difficulty with anxiety may be

TABLE 1.7 — TYPES OF DELUSIONS

Delusion	Description
Ideas of reference	Conviction that there are "meanings" behind events, media, and people's actions that are directed specifically toward oneself
Delusions of influence	Belief that one can control events through telepathy or other means
Persecutory delusions	Belief that one is being tormented, followed, tricked, spied on, or subjected to ridicule
Thought broadcasting	Belief that others can hear or read one's thoughts
Thought insertion	Belief that someone else's thoughts have been inserted into one's mind
Bizarre delusions	Belief involving a phenomenon that the person's culture would regard as totally implausible
Grandiose delusions	Feelings of inflated worth, power, talents, knowledge, identity, importance, or special relationship with famous people or a deity
Somatic delusions	Belief concerning the appearance or functioning of one's body
Ergotomatic delusions	Belief that another person, usually of higher status, is in love with one
Derealization	Perception of the world as unreal
Depersonalization	Feeling of removal from the reality of one's body
Lack of insight	Unawareness of illness or need for treatment even though it is evident to others

1

TABLE 1.8 — CHARACTERISTICS OF FORMAL THOUGHT DISORDER

Loosening of associations	Disconnected ideas and jumping from topic to unconnected topic
Neologisms	Coining new words (may have symbolic meaning)
Tangentiality	Abandoning one's ideational objective in pursuit of thoughts peripheral to the original goal
Word salad	Displaying an incomprehensible mixture of words and phrases
Overinclusiveness	Disruption of the flow of thoughts by inclusion of irrelevant information
Thought blocking	Halting of speech, often in mid-sentence, which is then picked up later, usually at another point in the thought process
Clanging	Selection of words and themes based on the sound of the words used rather than on thought content
Echolalia	Repetition of words or phrases in a musical or singsong fashion but without an apparent effort to communicate
Concreteness	Poor ability to think in abstract terms, despite normal or above average intelligence quotient (IQ)
Circumstantiality	Giving an extensive description of insignificant detail before eventually arriving at the original goal
Perseveration	Repeating a response to varied stimuli

TABLE 1.9 — NEGATIVE SYMPTOMS	
Symptoms	**Description**
Alogia	Speaking very little but without being intentionally resistant (poverty of speech) or may speak a normal amount but say very little (poverty of speech content)
Anhedonia	Loss of joy and interest in activities
Avolition	Inability to initiate and persist in goal-directed activities; may prevent one from completing activities
Blunted affect	Facial appearance that is immobile and unresponsive, with poor eye contact and reduced body language
Poor social skills	Diminished social involvement associated with unwarranted fear, hostility, distrust, apathy, or passivity
Poor grooming	Neglect and apathy concerning appearance and hygiene

exhibited due to positive symptoms and suspiciousness. Patients may have impaired self-care skills and may be dirty and unkempt due to negative symptoms. Sleep and appetite are often disturbed. Patients often have difficulty living independently in the community and have difficulty forming close relationships with others. Additionally, such patients have problems with initiating or maintaining employment and are often nonadherent with medications, thereby increasing their risk for relapse.

Diagnosis

The commonly accepted diagnostic criteria for schizophrenia come from the *Diagnostic and Statistical Manual of Mental Disorders*, 4th edition (DSM-

IV). The essential features are a mixture of characteristic signs and symptoms as listed above that have been present for a significant portion of time during a 1-month period (or a shorter time if successfully treated), with some signs of the disorder persisting for at least 6 months. These signs and symptoms are:

- Associated with marked social or occupational dysfunction
- Not accounted for by a mood disorder
- Not due to the direct physiologic effects of a substance or a general medical condition (Table 1.10)

There are subtypes of schizophrenia that are defined by predominant symptomatology at the time of evaluation. The clinical picture present at the most recent evaluation or admission is the subtype usually given to categorize the patient and may, therefore, change over time. Not infrequently, the presentation may include symptoms that are characteristic of more than one subtype. The subtypes are assigned according to the following categories:

- *Catatonic type* is whenever prominent catatonic symptoms are present (regardless of the presence of other symptoms).
- *Disorganized type* is assigned whenever disorganization of speech and behavior and flat or inappropriate affect are prominent.
- *Paranoid type* is assigned whenever there is a preoccupation with delusions or frequent hallucinations.
- *Undifferentiated type* is a category describing presentations that include prominent active-phase symptoms not meeting other types.
- *Residual type* is assigned to presentations in which there is continuing evidence of the disturbance, but the criteria for the active-phase symptoms are no longer met.

Differential diagnosis of psychotic signs and symptoms is shown in Table 1.11.

Course and Prognosis

Although the course of schizophrenia is variable, the long-term prognosis for independent function is often poor. This illness is marked by intermittent acute psychotic episodes and a downward decline in psychosocial functioning. A patient may become more withdrawn, bizarre, and nonfunctional over many years. Complete return to full premorbid functioning is not common in this disorder. Many of the more dramatic and acute symptoms will disappear with time, but severe residual symptoms may persist. Family and friends may find this illness difficult to interpret and understand. Involvement with the law is fairly common for misdemeanors such as vagrancy, loitering, and disturbing the peace. The overall life expectancy is shortened primarily due to suicide, accidents, and the inability for self-care. The lifetime risk of suicide for patients with schizophrenia is 10% to 13%, with an incidence of 350 to 600/100,000 compared with 11/100,000 in the general population. Patients who have fewer periods of acute psychotic episodes and those who are treated early in their course of illness may have a better prognosis. Persistent adherence to a tolerable drug regimen also improves prognosis (Table 1.12). Some symptoms will respond better to treatment than others (Figure 1.2).

The natural history of antipsychotic-treated schizophrenia is poorly understood, since traditional antipsychotics tended to cause many side effects that markedly lessened adherence and increased the incidence of negative symptoms in chronic patients. It remains to be seen whether the SGADs will offer better outcomes in the long term; however, based on their first 5 years of use in the clinical setting, there is much

TABLE 1.10 — DIAGNOSTIC CRITERIA FOR SCHIZOPHRENIA

A. *Characteristic Symptoms:* Two (or more) of the following, each present for a significant portion of time during a 1-month period (or less if successfully treated):

(1) Delusions
(2) Hallucinations
(3) Disorganized speech (eg, frequent derailment or incoherence)
(4) Grossly disorganized or catatonic behavior
(5) Negative symptoms, ie, affective flattening, alogia, or avolition

NOTE: Only one Criterion A symptom is required if delusions are bizarre or hallucinations consist of a voice keeping up a running commentary on the person's behavior or thoughts, or two or more voices conversing with each other.

B. *Social/Occupational Dysfunction:* For a significant portion of the time since the onset of the disturbance, one or more major areas of functioning such as work, interpersonal relations, or self-care are markedly below the level achieved prior to the onset (or when the onset is in childhood or adolescence, failure to achieve expected level of interpersonal, academic, or occupational achievement).

C. *Duration:* Continuous signs of the disturbance persist for at least 6 months. This 6-month period must include at least 1 month of symptoms (or less if successfully treated) that meet Criterion A (ie, active-phase symptoms) and may include periods of prodromal or residual symptoms. During these prodromal or residual periods, the signs of the disturbance may be manifested by only negative symptoms or two or more symptoms listed in Criterion A present in an attenuated form (eg, odd beliefs, unusual perceptual experiences).

D. *Schizoaffective and Mood Disorder Exclusion:* Schizoaffective disorder and mood disorder with psychotic features have been ruled out because either:
  (1) No major depressive, manic, or mixed episodes have occurred concurrently with the active-phase symptoms; or
  (2) If mood episodes have occurred during active-phase symptoms, their total duration has been brief relative to the duration of the active and residual periods.

E. *Substance/General Medical Condition Exclusion:* The disturbance is not due to the direct physiologic effects of a substance (eg, a drug of abuse, a medication) or a general medical condition.

F. *Relationship to a Pervasive Developmental Disorder:* If there is a history of autistic disorder or another pervasive developmental disorder, the additional diagnosis of schizophrenia is made only if prominent delusions or hallucinations are also present for at least 1 month (or less if successfully treated).

Classification of Longitudinal Course (can be applied only after at least 1 year has elapsed since the initial onset of active-phase symptoms):
  • *Episodic With Interepisode Residual Symptoms* (episodes are defined by the reemergence of prominent psychotic symptoms); also specify if:
  With Prominent Negative Symptoms
  • *Episodic With No Interepisode Residual Symptoms*
  • *Continuous* (prominent psychotic symptoms are present throughout the period of observation); also specify if: *With Prominent Negative Symptoms*
  • *Single Episode in Partial Remission*; also specify if: *With Prominent Negative Symptoms*
  • *Single Episode in Full Remission*
  • *Other or Unspecified Pattern*

American Psychiatric Association. *Diagnostic and Statistical Manual of Mental Disorders.* 4th ed. Washington, DC: American Psychiatric Press; 1994.

TABLE 1.11 — DIFFERENTIAL DIAGNOSIS OF PSYCHOTIC SIGNS AND SYMPTOMS

- Schizoaffective disorder
- Mood disorder
- Dementia
- Delirium
- Drug intoxication
- Pervasive developmental disorder
- Neurologic conditions (neoplasms, migraines, Huntington's chorea, deafness, epilepsy)
- Metabolic conditions (hypoxia, hypercapnia, hypoglycemia)
- Endocrine conditions (hyperthyroidism, hypothyroidism, hyperparathyroidism, hypoparathyroidism, hypoadrenocorticism)
- Fluid or electrolyte imbalances
- Hepatic or renal disease
- Autoimmune disorders
- Hypnagogic and hypnopompic hallucinations

TABLE 1.12 — CLINICAL CHARACTERISTICS ASSOCIATED WITH AN IMPROVED PROGNOSIS

- No family history of schizophrenia
- Rapid onset of active psychotic symptoms
- Good premorbid social and occupational functioning
- Probable precipitating stress to the acute psychosis
- No evidence of central nervous system abnormalities
- Marriage
- Paranoid subtype
- Later onset of illness
- Early temporal treatment in the course of illness

cause for hope. The order of responsiveness of symptoms may change as the number of patients treated with SGADs increases.

FIGURE 1.2 — RESPONSIVENESS OF SYMPTOMS

Most Responsive

Combativeness and hostility

Tension and hyperactivity

Hallucinations

Sleep

Appetite

Hygiene and dress

Delusions

Judgment

Social skills

Affect

Insight

Amotivation

Diminished speech

Content of speech

Social inadequacy

Least Responsive

SUGGESTED READING

American Psychiatric Association. *Diagnostic and Statistical Manual of Mental Disorders*. 4th ed. (DSM-IV). Washington, DC: American Psychiatric Press, Inc; 1994.

Andreasen NC, Carpenter WT Jr. Diagnosis and classification of schizophrenia. *Schizophr Bull*. 1993;19:199-214.

Carlsson A, Waters N, Carlsson ML. Neurotransmitter interactions in schizophrenia—therapeutic implications. *Biol Psychiatry*. 1999; 46:1388-1395.

Farber NB, Newcomer JW, Olney JW. The glutamate synapse in neuropsychiatric disorders. Focus on schizophrenia and Alzheimer's disease. *Prog Brain Res*. 1998;116:421-437.

Gelman S. *Medicating Schizophrenia: A History*. New Brunswick, NJ and London, UK: Rutgers University Press; 1999.

Martin MB, Owen CM, Morihisa JM. An overview of neurotransmitters and neuroceptors. In: Hales RE, Yudofsky SC, eds. *Textbook of Neuropsychiatry*. Washington DC: American Psychiatric Press; 1997:55-85.

McClure RJ, Keshavan MS, Pettegrew JW. Chemical and physiologic brain imaging in schizophrenia. *Psychiatr Clin North Am*. 1998;21:93-122.

Pearlson GD, Marsh L. Structural brain imaging in schizophrenia: a selective review. *Biol Psychiatry*. 1999;46:627-649.

Tsuang MT, Stone WS, Faraone SV. Schizophrenia: a review of genetic studies. *Harv Rev Psychiatry*. 1999;7:185-207.

2   Treatment of Schizophrenia

History

Antipsychotic drugs are used to treat nearly all forms of psychosis, including:

- Schizophrenia
- Schizoaffective disorder
- Affective disorders with psychosis
- Dementias.

The first antipsychotic drugs available, the traditional or conventional antipsychotics as termed in this book, were previously referred to as neuroleptic agents. These drugs all have important limitations to their use:

- They are not effective in all patients.
- They have several serious adverse effects.
- They have a history of poor long-term outcomes associated with their use.

These limitations have prompted a search for newer medications with better side effect profiles and improved effectiveness.

Chlorpromazine was the first conventional antipsychotic available. This drug was initially developed for controlling preoperative anxiety, but within its first year of use it was recognized as a potential treatment for psychosis. This medication gained rapid acceptance due to the lack of other effective treatments for psychosis. Many other medications, such as thioridazine, fluphenazine, haloperidol, and thiothixene, were marketed shortly thereafter. The second-generation antipsychotic drugs (SGADs) (atypical or novel antipsychotics) were first introduced in the late 1980s, with the prototypical agent, clozapine. This class of medication differed primarily by producing minimal or no extrapyramidal symptoms in humans and no catalepsy (defined as immobility for 20 seconds) in rodents. These agents treat a broader spectrum of symptoms of schizophrenia as compared with traditional agents.

Available Antipsychotic Drugs

This chapter will cover the available antipsychotic medications and their place in therapy. Chapter 3, *Second-Generation Antipsychotic Drugs,* and Chapter 5, *Conventional Antipsychotic Drugs,* will cover each class of medication more thoroughly. The available antipsychotics are listed in Table 2.1. More specific details on dosing and available preparations are located in the next chapters.

Treatment Recommendations

Traditional antipsychotics were considered the gold standard for treatment prior to the advent of novel antipsychotics. Despite their numerous advantages, however, the SGADs have not routinely moved into first-line therapy for all patients. This primarily has been due to two reasons:
- Novel agents lack the neuroleptic or tranquilizing effect that many clinicians were accustomed to and relied upon for initial therapy.
- The cost of newer medications is higher than the cost of traditional agents.

In early 2002 in the United States, 33% of patients were taking risperidone, 31% olanzapine, 12% quetiapine, 4% clozapine, and 3% ziprasidone, and traditional antipsychotics accounted for about 18% of all antipsychotics being used. Over the past several years, the number of patients on traditional agents has been rapidly diminishing. In 1997 and 1999, approximately 60% and 36% of patients, respectively, were taking traditional agents, while the use of SGADs has been increasing. Clinicians are realizing the benefits of atypical drugs as compared with traditional antipsychotics and are utilizing benzodiazepines and other strategies for acute treatment and agitation (see Chapter 8, *Management of Acute Psychosis, Psychiatric Emergencies, and Aggressive/Suicidal Behavior*). Additionally, accumulating evidence suggests that despite the higher cost of SGADs, these medications are more cost-effective than traditional agents (see Chapter 15, *Outcomes and Health-Services Research*). Thus SGADs (not including clozapine) are now considered to be first-line therapy for most patients with schizophrenia.

Treatment recommendations have been developed through the use of consensus guidelines and algorithms. Some medication recommendations from the Schizophrenia Patient Outcomes Research Team project are listed in Table 2.2. The Texas Medication Algorithm Project (TMAP) recommends SGAD use as first-line treatment in people with schizophrenia.

The most recent set of treatment guidelines comes from the Expert Consensus Guidelines for the Treatment of Schizophrenia, which was published by the *Journal of Clinical Psychiatry* in 1999. These guidelines are based on information from leaders in the field of psychiatric research concerning standards of practice for the treatment of schizophrenia, yet unfortunately do not include newer antipsychotic drugs, such as ziprasidone and aripiprazole. Table 2.3 lists recommendations for antipsychotic use in specific situations.

Rating Scales

Unlike many other branches of medicine, psychiatry—and specifically the treatment of schizophrenia—

TABLE 2.1 — AVAILABLE ANTIPSYCHOTIC DRUGS FOR THE TREATMENT OF SCHIZOPHRENIA

Generic Name	Trade Name	Manufacturer	Conventional Equivalent Dose (mg)
Conventional Antipsychotic Drugs			
Chlorpromazine	Thorazine, others	GlaxoSmithKline, others	100
Fluphenazine	Many	Many	2
Haloperidol	Haldol, others	Ortho-McNeil, others	2
Loxapine	Loxitane	Watson	10
Mesoridazine	Serentil	Boehringer Ingelheim	50
Molindone	Moban	Endo	10
Perphenazine	Trilafon, others	Schering, others	10
Pimozide	Orap	Gate	1
Thioridazine	Many	Many	100
Thiothixene	Navane, others	Pfizer, others	4
Trifluoperazine	Stelazine, others	GlaxoSmithKline, others	5

Second-Generation Antipsychotic Drugs*		
Aripiprazole	Abilify	Otsuka	6-7
Clozapine	Clozaril, others	Novartis, others	50
Olanzapine	Zyprexa	Lilly	4-5
Quetiapine	Seroquel	AstraZeneca	50
Risperidone	Risperdal	Janssen	1
Ziprasidone	Geodon	Pfizer	20

* Second-generation antipsychotic drugs, unlike conventional agents, do not have clinical dose ranges that can be easily predicted from *in vitro* activity. The "dose equivalents" given here are approximate and based on clinical observation.

TABLE 2.2 — SCHIZOPHRENIA TREATMENT RECOMMENDATIONS

- Antipsychotic medications other than clozapine should be used as the first-line treatment to reduce psychotic symptoms in persons experiencing an acute-symptom episode of schizophrenia.
- The dose of antipsychotic medication for an acute-symptom episode should be in the range of 300 to 1,000 chlorpromazine (CPZ) equivalents per day for a minimum of 6 weeks.* Reasons for doses outside this range should be justified and the minimal effective dose should be used.
- Prophylactic use of antiparkinsonian agents to reduce the incidence of extrapyramidal symptoms (EPS) should be determined on a case-by-case basis, taking into account patient and physician preferences, prior individual history of EPS, and other risk factors for both EPS and anticholinergic side effects. The effectiveness of and continued need for antiparkinsonian agents should be assessed in an ongoing fashion.
- Persons who experience acute-symptom relief with an antipsychotic medication should continue to receive this medication for at least 1 year subsequent to symptom stabilization to reduce the risk of relapse or worsening of positive symptoms.
- The maintenance dose of antipsychotic medication should be in the range of 300 to 600 CPZ equivalents (oral or depot) per day.*
- Depot antipsychotic maintenance therapy should be strongly considered in persons who have difficulty complying with an oral medication regimen or who prefer the depot regimen.
- Persons who experience persistent and clinically significant associated symptoms of anxiety, depression, or hostility, despite an adequate reduction in positive symptoms with antipsychotic therapy, should receive a trial of adjunctive pharmacotherapy.

- Persons who experience persistent and clinically significant positive symptoms despite adequate antipsychotic therapy, including trials with newer antipsychotics, should receive a trial of adjunctive pharmacotherapy.

* This dose range was based on the use of conventional antipsychotics and cannot be exactly translated into an appropriate dose for second-generation antipsychotic drugs.

Lehman AF, Steinwachs DM. *Schizophr Bull.* 1998;24:11-20.

lacks laboratory or other biologic measures that can be used to assess the presence and severity of disease, or the response to treatment. Objective rating scales to assess a wide variety of symptoms and side effects exist to help both the clinician and the researcher determine how a patient is doing. Several rating scales are used in assessing the treatment of schizophrenia.

Efficacy Measures

■ Brief Psychiatric Rating Scale
The Brief Psychiatric Rating Scale is an 18-item scale that measures major symptoms, both psychotic and nonpsychotic (Figure 2.1). It is appropriate for assessing baseline psychopathology, clinical course, and treatment response. This instrument is rated on a 7-point scale (1 = not present, 7 = very severe). This scale is probably the most widely used scale in the assessment of schizophrenia treatment and has been found to be reliable. A 20% decrease in symptoms is often used as a standard of response on this rating scale.

■ Clinical Global Impression
The Clinical Global Impression is a 3-item scale that assesses treatment response in psychiatric patients. It is used to monitor clinical course and may be ad-

TABLE 2.3 — RECOMMENDATIONS FOR ANTIPSYCHOTIC USE IN SPECIFIC SITUATIONS

- First-episode schizophrenic patients with predominately positive symptoms should be treated with second-generation antipsychotic drugs (SGADs) as first-line therapy
- The recommended antipsychotics for persistent aggression and violence are clozapine and high-potency traditional agents
- Recommended antipsychotics in patients with insomnia include SGADs and low-potency traditional agents
- SGADs are preferred over conventional agents in patients with:
  - Comorbid substance abuse
  - Dysphoria
  - Cognitive problems
- Clozapine is the preferred agent in patients who exhibit excessive water drinking
- Risperidone, ziprasidone, or aripiprazole is preferred in patients when sedation should be avoided
- Risperidone, quetiapine, ziprasidone, or aripiprazole is preferred in patients when weight gain should be avoided
- SGADs should be used in patients when extrapyramidal symptoms should be avoided.
- Risperidone, quetiapine, ziprasidone, aripiprazole, and high-potency agents should be used in patients when anticholinergic effects should be avoided
- Quetiapine, ziprasidone, aripiprazole, or clozapine should be used in patients when sexual/reproductive side effects should be avoided

ministered to many diagnostic groups of patients. The three items include:
- Severity of illness
- Global improvement
- Efficacy index.

Item 1 is rated on a 7-point scale (1 = normal, 7 = among the most extremely ill patients), as is item

2 (1 = very much improved, 7 = very much worse). Item 3 is rated on a 4-point scale (from "none" to "outweighs therapeutic effects"). The brevity of the scale, its simplicity, and its high validity are all favorable aspects of this scale. This scale is easily used in routine clinical care.

■ Positive and Negative Syndrome Scale

The Positive and Negative Syndrome Scale (PANSS) is a 30-item rating scale that assesses positive, negative, and other symptoms in patients with schizophrenia. The instrument is rated on a 7-point scale (1 = absent, 7 = extreme). Seven items each are grouped to form a positive scale and a negative scale. High inter-rater reliability and test-retest reliability have been demonstrated for the scale. Additionally, the PANSS shows a close correspondence with the Scale for the Assessment of Negative Symptoms and the Scale for the Assessment of Positive Symptoms.

■ Global Assessment Scale

The Global Assessment Scale (GAS) is a single-item rating scale for evaluating overall functioning of a subject during a specified period (Figure 2.2). The period assessed is usually the week prior to administration. The scoring ranges from 1 to 100, with 100 being the healthiest individual to 1, the most ill. The Global Assessment of Functioning (GAF) scale, which is used for rating Axis V of the *Diagnostic and Statistical Manual of Mental Disorders*, 4th edition, is a revision of the GAS. The GAF has slightly differing anchor points and does not include individuals with superior functioning. A score of 100 on the GAF equates to normal functioning with no symptoms.

FIGURE 2.1 — BRIEF PSYCHIATRIC RATING SCALE

Subject _____

Rater _____

Date _____

	NOT PRESENT	VERY MILD	MILD	MODERATE	MODERATE-SEVERE	SEVERE	VERY SEVERE	NOT ASSESSED
1. *Somatic Concern*—Degree of concern over present bodily health. Rate the degree to which physical health is perceived as a problem by the patient, whether complaints have a realistic basis or not.	1	2	3	4	5	6	7	8
2. *Anxiety*—Worry, fear, or overconcern for present or future. Rate solely on the basis of verbal report of patient's own subjective experiences. Do not infer anxiety from physical signs of neurotic defense mechanisms.	1	2	3	4	5	6	7	8
3. *Emotional Withdrawal*—Deficiency in relating to the interviewer and to the interview situation. Rate only the degree to which the patient gives the impression of failing to be in emotional contact with other people in the interview situation.	1	2	3	4	5	6	7	8
4. *Conceptual Disorganization*—Degree to which the thought processes are confused, disconnected, or disorganized. Rate only on the basis of integration of the verbal products of the patient; do not rate on the basis of the patient's subjective impression of his own level of functioning.	1	2	3	4	5	6	7	8

	1	2	3	4	5	6	7	8
5. *Guilt Feelings*—Overconcern or remorse for past behavior. Rate on the basis of the patient's subjective experiences of guilt as evidenced by verbal report with appropriate affect; do not infer guilt feelings from depression, anxiety, or neurotic defenses.	1	2	3	4	5	6	7	8
6. *Tension*—Physical and motor manifestations of tension, nervousness, and heightened activation level. Tension should be rated solely on the basis of physical signs and motor behavior and not on the basis of subjective experiences of tension reported by the patient.	1	2	3	4	5	6	7	8
7. *Mannerisms and Posturing*—Unusual and unnatural motor behavior, the type of motor behavior that causes certain mental patients to stand out in a crowd of normal people. Rate only abnormality of movements; do not rate simple heightened motor activity. Do not rate movements of tardive dyskinesia.	1	2	3	4	5	6	7	8
8. *Grandiosity*—Exaggerated self-opinion, conviction of unusual ability, or powers. Rate only on the basis of patient's statements about self or self in relation to others, not on the basis of demeanor in the interview situation.	1	2	3	4	5	6	7	8
9. *Depressive Mood*—Despondency in mood, sadness. Rate only degree of despondency; do not rate on the basis of inferences concerning depression based upon general retardation and somatic complaints.	1	2	3	4	5	6	7	8

Continued

2

Subject _____

Rater _____

Date _____

	Not Present	Very Mild	Mild	Moderate	Moderate-Severe	Severe	Very Severe	Not Assessed
10. *Hostility*—Animosity, contempt, belligerence, disdain for other people outside the interview situation. Rate solely on the basis of the verbal report of feelings and actions of the patient toward others; do not infer hostility from neurotic defenses, anxiety, or somatic complaints. (Rate attitude toward interviewer under "uncooperativeness.")	1	2	3	4	5	6	7	8
11. *Suspiciousness*—Belief (delusional or otherwise) that others have now, or have had in the past, malicious or discriminatory intent toward the patient. On the basis of verbal report, rate only those suspicions that are currently held, whether they concern past or present circumstances.	1	2	3	4	5	6	7	8
12. *Hallucinatory Behavior*—Perceptions without normal external stimulus correspondence. Rate only those experiences that are reported to have occurred within the last week and which are described as distinctly different from the thought and imagery processes of normal people.	1	2	3	4	5	6	7	8

	1	2	3	4	5	6	7	8
13. *Motor Retardation*—Reduction in energy level evidenced in slowed movements. Rate on the basis of observed behavior of the patient only; do not rate on the basis of patient's subjective impression of own energy level.	1	2	3	4	5	6	7	8
14. *Uncooperativeness*—Evidence of resistance, unfriendliness, resentment, and lack of readiness to cooperate with the interviewer. Rate only on the basis of the patient's attitude and responses to the interviewer and the interview situation; do not rate on the basis of reported resentment or uncooperativeness outside the interview situation.	1	2	3	4	5	6	7	8
15. *Unusual Thought Content*—Unusual, odd, strange, or bizarre thought content. Rate here the degree of unusualness, not the degree of disorganization of thought process.	1	2	3	4	5	6	7	8
16. *Blunted Affect*—Reduced emotional tone, apparent lack of normal feeling or involvement.	1	2	3	4	5	6	7	8
17. *Excitement*—Heightened emotional tone, agitation, increased reactivity.	1	2	3	4	5	6	7	8
18. *Disorientation*—Confusion or lack of proper association for person, place, or time.	1	2	3	4	5	6	7	8

FIGURE 2.2 — GLOBAL ASSESSMENT SCALE

Rate the patient's lowest level of functioning in the last week by selecting the *lowest range* that describes his/her functioning on a hypothetical continuum of mental illness. For example, a patient whose "behavior is considerably influenced by delusions" (range 21-30) should be given a rating in that range even though he/she has "major impairment in several areas" (range 31-40). Use intermediary levels when appropriate (eg, 35, 58, 63). Rate actual functioning *independent* of whether or not patient is receiving and may be helped by medication or some other form of treatment.

_____ (100–91)	No symptoms, superior functioning in a wide range of activities, life's problems never seem to get out of hand, is sought out by others because of his/her warmth and integrity.
_____ (90–81)	Transient symptoms may occur, but good functioning in all areas, interested and involved in a wide range of activities, socially effective, generally satisfied with life, "everyday" worries only occasionally get out of hand.
_____ (80–71)	Minimal symptoms may be present but no more than slight impairment in functioning, varying degrees of "everyday" worries and problems that sometimes get out of hand.
_____ (70–61)	Some mild symptoms (eg, depressive mood and mild insomnia) OR some difficulty in several areas of functioning, but generally functioning pretty well, has some meaningful interpersonal relationships and most untrained people would not consider him/her "sick."

____ (60-51)	Moderate symptoms OR generally functioning with some difficulty (eg, few friends and flat affect, depressed mood, and pathologic self-doubt, euphoric mood and pressure of speech, moderately severe antisocial behavior).
____ (50-41)	Any serious symptomatology or impairment in functioning that most clinicians would think obviously requires treatment or attention (eg, suicidal preoccupation or gesture, severe obsessional rituals, frequent anxiety attacks, serious antisocial behavior, compulsive drinking).
____ (40-31)	Major impairment in several areas, such as work, family relations, judgment, thinking, or mood (eg, depressed woman avoids friends, neglects family, unable to do housework) OR some impairment in reality testing or communication (eg, speech is at times obscure, illogical, or irrelevant) OR single serious suicide attempt.
____ (30-21)	Unable to function in almost all areas (eg, stays in bed all day) OR behavior is considerably influenced by either delusions or hallucinations OR serious impairment in communication (eg, sometimes incoherent or unresponsive) or judgment (eg, acts grossly inappropriately).
____ (20-11)	Needs some supervision to prevent hurting self and others or to maintain minimal personal hygiene (eg, repeated suicide attempts, frequently violent, manic excitement, smears feces) OR gross impairment in communication (eg, largely incoherent or mute).
____ (10-1)	Needs constant supervision for several days to prevent hurting self or others or makes no attempt to maintain personal hygiene.

Side Effect Scales

The three most widely used rating instruments for side effects in patients treated with antipsychotics include:

- Simpson-Angus Scale (SAS)
- Abnormal Involuntary Movement Scale (AIMS)
- Barnes Akathisia Rating Scale (BARS).

The SAS is a 10-item instrument used to measure drug-induced parkinsonism by assessing rigidity, tremor, and salivation. It is rated on a 5-point scale (0 = complete absence of the condition, 4 = presence of the condition in extreme form). The AIMS is a 12-item instrument that assesses abnormal involuntary movements, specifically tardive dyskinesia, related to antipsychotic therapy. Scoring of the AIMS examination consists of rating the severity of movements in three main areas: facial/oral, extremities, and trunk. This instrument is based on a 5-point scale (0 = none, 4 = severe). The BARS is a 4-item scale used to assess drug-induced akathisia. This scale evaluates objective and subjective features of restlessness and associated distress, which are rated from 0 to 3. There is also a global severity rating on a 6-point scale (0 = absent, 5 = severe). A rating of 2 or more is considered diagnostic for akathisia.

SUGGESTED READING

Kane JM. Pharmacologic treatment of schizophrenia. *Biol Psychiatry*. 1999;46:1396-1408.

Lehman AF. Improving treatment for persons with schizophrenia. *Psychiatr Q*. 1999;70:259-272.

Lehman AF, Steinwachs DM. Patterns of usual care for schizophrenia: initial results for the Schizophrenia Patient Outcomes Research Team (PORT) Client Survey. *Schizophr Bull*. 1998;24:11-20.

Remington G, Chong SA. Conventional versus novel antipsychotics: changing concepts and clinical implications. *J Psychiatry Neurosci*. 1999;24:431-441.

Shen WW. A history of antipsychotic drug development. *Compr Psychiatry*. 1999;40:407-414.

Treatment of schizophrenia 1999. The expert consensus guideline series. *J Clin Psychiatry*. 1999;60(suppl 11):3-80.

2

3

Second-Generation Antipsychotic Drugs

While conventional or traditional antipsychotics exert most of their receptor blockade through dopamine-2 (D_2) receptors, the second-generation antipsychotic drugs (SGADs) may work through different mechanisms. The latter agents have greater affinity for serotonin receptors than for dopamine receptors. The involvement of serotonin in the mechanism of action of SGADs was postulated partly because serotonin is known to exert a regulatory action on dopamine neurons. Studies suggest that serotonin projections inhibit mesolimbic and nigrostriatal dopaminergic activity and may directly inhibit dopamine release from striatal nerve terminals. The antipsychotic drug profiles for receptor binding are shown in Figure 3.1.

These medications as a class, however, are heterogeneous in regards to receptor binding and structure activity. The chemical structures for the SGADs are shown in Figure 3.2. The structures of olanzapine and quetiapine are similar to the dibenzodiazepine structure of clozapine. These medications, however, do not possess the superior efficacy of clozapine. Risperidone and ziprasidone are similar in structure but very different from the other available SGADs. While aripiprazole has a very different structure from the other SGADs and a unique pharmacologic mechanism of action, this SGAD is the first antipsychotic drug to function as a D_2 partial agonist rather than a D_2 antagonist.

The SGADs and a summary of dosing information are provided in Table 3.1. Information on the SGADs in regard to mechanism of action, efficacy, dosing, pharmacokinetics, and adverse effects follows.

FIGURE 3.1 — ANTIPSYCHOTIC DRUG PROFILES FOR RECEPTOR BINDING

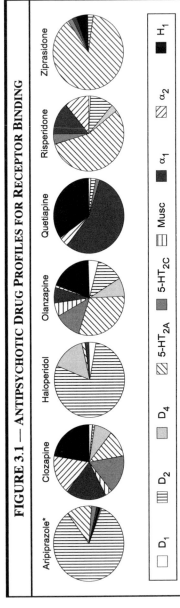

Abbreviations: D, dopamine; 5-HT, serotonin; Musc, muscarinic; H, histamine.

* Partial agonist activity at D_2 receptors, whereas all others are D_2 antagonists; muscarinic <0.01%; also has D_3 activity.

Adapted from: Collaborative Working Group on Clinical Evaluations. *J Clin Psychiatry.* 1998;59(suppl 12):7. Data on file for aripiprazole: Otsuka America Pharmaceutical, Inc., Rockville, Md.

FIGURE 3.2 — CHEMICAL STRUCTURES OF SECOND-GENERATION ANTIPSYCHOTIC DRUGS COMPARED WITH HALOPERIDOL

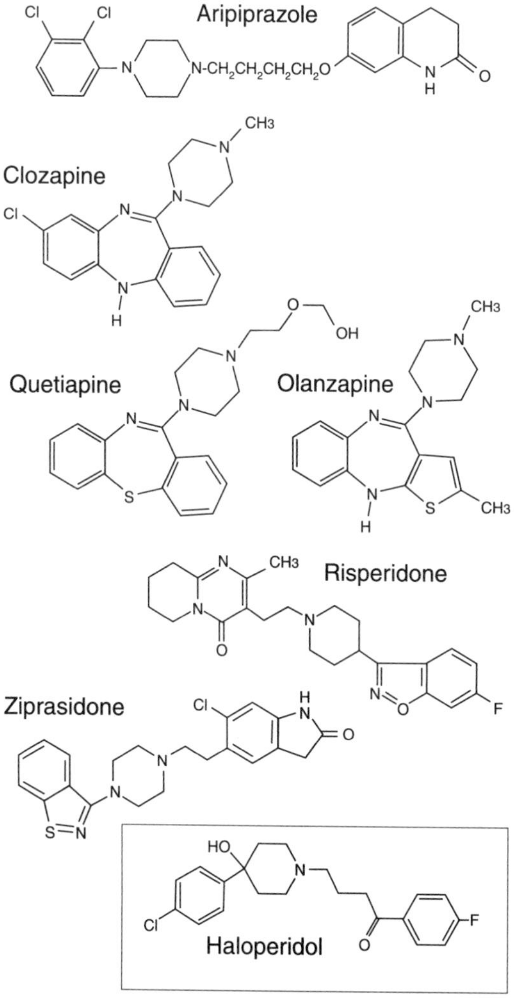

Aripiprazole

Clozapine

Quetiapine

Olanzapine

Risperidone

Ziprasidone

Haloperidol

TABLE 3.1 — SUMMARY OF DOSING INFORMATION FOR SECOND-GENERATION ANTIPSYCHOTIC DRUGS		
Antipsychotic Drug	**Usual Dosage Range** (mg/d)	**Available Dosage Forms**
Aripiprazole	10-30	10-, 15-, 20-, and 30-mg tablets
Clozapine	300-700	25- and 100-mg tablets
Olanzapine	10-20	2.5-, 5-, 7.5-, 10-, 15-, and 20-mg tablets; Zyprexa Zydis: 5-, 10-, 15-, and 20-mg orally disintegrating tablets
Quetiapine	300-800	25-, 100-, 200-, and 300-mg tablets
Risperidone	2-6	0.25-, 0.5-, 1-, 2-, 3-, and 4-mg tablets; 1 mg/mL (30 mL) oral solution
Ziprasidone	40-160	20-, 40-, 60-, and 80-mg capsules; ziprasidone mesylate IM 20 mg/mL

Abbreviation: IM, intramuscular.

Comparative data are presented in Chapter 4, *Comparative Data Among Second-Generation Antipsychotic Drugs*, and information on extrapyramidal symptoms (EPS) and tardive dyskinesia is listed in Chapter 6, *Extrapyramidal Symptoms/Tardive Dyskinesia*. Adverse effects in clinical trials occurring with the greatest frequency are listed as well as additional information on other clinically significant or controversial side effects.

Aripiprazole

■ History and Mechanism of Action

Aripiprazole was discovered in the late 1980s in an attempt to find an antipsychotic drug that would function as a potential entity with both antagonist and agonist activity to the D_2 receptor. *In vitro* data suggested that the dopamine autoreceptor agonists were effective in treating negative symptoms of schizophrenia. Potent dopamine postsynaptic receptor antagonism was believed to be necessary for positive symptoms of schizophrenia. Hence, aripiprazole is the first potent D_2 partial agonist for the treatment of schizophrenia. In a hyperdopaminergic state, aripiprazole functions as an antagonist, while under conditions of hypodopaminergic activity, it functions more like an agonist. This novel mechanism has been labeled a dopamine system stabilizer and provides efficacy comparable to other antipsychotic drugs with minimal incidence of serious adverse effects. Aripiprazole also has high affinity for D_3 receptors. It is also a partial agonist at the $5\text{-}HT_{1A}$ receptor and an antagonist at the $5\text{-}HT_{2A}$ receptor. Aripiprazole has moderate affinity for the alpha-1 (α_1) and H_1 receptors with no appreciable affinity for the M_1 receptor.

■ Efficacy

The efficacy of aripiprazole was demonstrated in four short-term (4 to 6 weeks), placebo-controlled trials in patients with schizophrenia or schizoaffective disorder. Three phase III pivotal trials were performed with one each including haloperidol and risperidone. The first trial found both the 15- and 30-mg/day dose to be superior to placebo and similar to haloperidol compared with placebo. The second trial found 20 and 30 mg to be superior to placebo and similar to risperidone compared with placebo. A third trial also found 10, 15, and 20 mg to be superior to placebo. Significant improvements were seen for all symptom domains such as Positive and Negative Syndrome Scale (PANSS) total, positive, and negative symptoms. Longer-term studies have shown maintenance of effect and relapse rates lower than those with placebo and similar to those with haloperidol.

■ Dosing

The recommended starting dose is 10 to 15 mg every day given without regard to meals. No titration is required since the starting dose is an effective dose for many individuals. Ten to 30 mg daily is recommended as the dosing range. Doses greater than 30 mg have not been systematically evaluated. Doses higher than 10 or 15 mg/day were not more effective than doses of 10 or 15 mg/day.

■ Pharmacokinetics

The pharmacokinetics of aripiprazole are dose proportional. Aripiprazole is well absorbed following oral administration. The mean elimination half-life is about 75 hours, which readily allows for once-daily dosing. Steady state is reached within 2 weeks.

TABLE 3.2 — ADVERSE EFFECTS OF ARIPIPRAZOLE COMPARED WITH PLACEBO

Side Effect	Aripiprazole (%)	Placebo (%)
Headache	32	25
Anxiety	25	24
Insomnia	24	19
Nausea	14	10
Vomiting	12	7
Somnolence	11	8
Light-headedness	11	7
Constipation	10	8
Akathisia	10	7
Asthenia	7	5
Rash	6	5
Rhinitis	4	3
Coughing	3	2
Tremor	3	2
Blurred vision	3	1
Fever	2	1

Data on file for aripiprazole: Otsuka America Pharmaceutical, Inc., Rockville, Md.

■ **Adverse Effects**

The adverse effects listed in Table 3.2 were spontaneously reported in the short-term, placebo-controlled trials and include only those events that occurred in 2% or more of patients treated with aripiprazole and for which the incidence in patients treated with aripiprazole was greater than in those treated with placebo. Overall rates of side effects were quite low. Sedation was the only side effect to have a possible dose-response relationship, and then it was most prominent only with the 30 mg dosage. Aripiprazole is associated with EPS similar to placebo and little to no effect on prolactin. Weight gain generally averages about 1 kg over 6-12 months. Data on EPS and prolactin effects can be found in Chapter 4, *Comparative Data Among Second-Generation Antipsychotic Drugs*.

Clozapine

■ History

Reports of clozapine being effective for psychosis first appeared in the mid 1960s. The use of this agent was controversial because clozapine did not produce EPS, which were thought to be required of an effective antipsychotic at that time. In the early 1970s, soon after clozapine began to be widely used, eight patients in Finland died from agranulocytosis while taking the drug. The use of clozapine declined until the late 1980s, when it reemerged as a treatment for a selected group of treatment-refractory patients. In 1990, after availability was for compassionate use only, clozapine was marketed in the United States. Therapeutic use now includes a weekly laboratory monitoring system.

■ Mechanism of Action

Clozapine is the only agent approved and effective for the treatment of therapy-refractory schizophrenia (see Chapter 11, *Treatment-Resistant Schizophrenia*). A great deal of interest has been generated in understanding what pharmacologic properties of clozapine contribute to its superior efficacy. Clozapine has an increased ratio of D_1 to D_2 antagonism, greater D_3 and D_4 blockade, 5-hydroxytryptamine (5-HT)$_{2A}$ and 5-HT$_{2C}$ antagonistic properties, anticholinergic and antiadrenergic properties, and increased meso-limbic specificity with relative sparing of nigrostriatal dopaminergic neurons.

■ Efficacy

Several trials have consistently found clozapine to be superior to traditional antipsychotics in treatment-refractory patients. Approximately 30% to 50% of patients with treatment-resistant schizophrenia are reported to respond to clozapine treatment. Kane and associates performed the landmark study that helped bring clozapine back into the armamentarium of treatments. His group compared clozapine with chlorpromazine in a stringent study design. Thirty percent of patients responded to clozapine while only 4% of those receiving chlorpromazine responded. Further discussion of treatment resistance can be found in Chapter 11, *Treatment-Resistant Schizophrenia.*

■ Dosing

Due to side effects such as orthostatic hypotension and sedation, titration is recommended for dosing (Table 3.3). Daily dosing should continue on a twice-daily regimen as an effective and tolerable dose level is sought. Most patients will respond to dosing between 300 and 600 mg/day. In a few instances, patients may respond to doses between 600 and 900 mg/day; however, this upper range is the maximum recommended dose. Doses higher than 600 mg/day are associated with an increased risk of adverse events,

TABLE 3.3 — DOSING RECOMMENDATIONS FOR CLOZAPINE	
Initiation	12.5 mg qd or bid
Titration	Increase by 25- to 50-mg/day increments
Target	300 to 450 mg/day by the end of 2 weeks

including seizures. Most patients who will benefit from clozapine will typically respond by the end of 8 weeks of therapy.

A consensus panel of the National Institute of Mental Health has recommended that if a patient is responding well to treatment with clozapine, withdrawal from the medication should be avoided unless it is medically warranted. Abrupt withdrawal of clozapine may lead to a rebound phenomenon, which may be attributed to the cholinergic component of clozapine. Cholinergic rebound after the withdrawal of medication typically is associated with somatic symptoms such as:

- Malaise
- Agitation
- Insomnia
- Restlessness
- Anorexia
- Nausea.

The propensity for the rapid onset of these withdrawal symptoms has been linked to the relatively short elimination half-life of clozapine and to the fact that it dissociates from its target receptors more rapidly than other antipsychotics. Aside from somatic symptoms, withdrawal from clozapine also may result in a recurrence of psychotic symptoms. If a patient has not taken clozapine for more than 2 days since the last dose, it is recommended that clozapine be reinitiated with 12.5 mg to 25 mg once or twice daily. If that dose is well tolerated, it may be feasible to titrate it to a therapeutic dose more quickly than is recommended for initial treatment. In patients who have previously experienced respiratory or cardiac complications with initial dosing, the dose should be retitrated with extreme caution after even 24 hours of discontinuation.

■ Pharmacokinetics

Clozapine is well absorbed (90% to 95%) and is not affected by the administration of food. It is 97% plasma protein bound and undergoes extensive first-pass metabolism, resulting in an oral bioavailability of about 50%. The major metabolite of clozapine is *N*-desmethylclozapine (norclozapine), an active metabolite with lower potency than the parent compound but one that may contribute to the bone marrow suppression. Clozapine is metabolized mostly by the cytochrome P450 (CYP450) enzyme 1A2, but 2D6 and 3A4 also play small roles in metabolism of this agent (see Chapter 13, *Drug Interactions With Antipsychotic Drugs*). The mean elimination half-life of clozapine after steady state dosing is 12 hours.

A clozapine dose of 300 mg/day at steady state will typically produce a plasma concentration between 200 and 600 ng/mL. Plasma concentrations above 350 ng/mL have been found to be associated with a greater likelihood of response.

■ Adverse Effects

The most frequently occurring side effects from clinical trials with clozapine are listed in Table 3.4. Information pertaining to treatment recommendations for anticholinergic effects can be found in Chapter 5, *Conventional Antipsychotic Drugs*.

Hematologic Side Effects

Current estimates are that agranulocytosis will develop in approximately 0.8% of patients treated with clozapine. Agranulocytosis is clinically defined as a granulocyte count of $<500/mm^3$, whereas neutropenia is defined as a neutrophil count of $<1000/mm^3$, and leukopenia, as a white blood cell (WBC) count of $<3500/mm^3$. The etiology of agranulocytosis is undetermined; however, it is believed to be immunologi-

TABLE 3.4 — ADVERSE EFFECTS OF CLOZAPINE*

Side Effect	Patients Experiencing Side Effect (%)
Drowsiness/sedation	39
Salivation	31
Tachycardia	25
Dizziness/vertigo	19
Constipation	14
Hypotension	9
Headache	7
Sweating	6
Dry mouth	6
Syncope	6
Tremor	6
Fever	5
Nausea	5
Visual disturbances	5
Abdominal discomfort/ heartburn	4
Agitation	4
Disturbed sleep/ nightmares	4
Hypertension	4
Hypokinesia/akinesia	4
Restlessness	4
Weight gain	4
Akathisia	3
Confusion	3
Leukopenia/decreased wbc/ neutropenia	3
Nausea/vomiting	3
Rigidity	3

Continued

Seizures	3
Vomiting	3
Diarrhea	2
Fatigue	2
Insomnia	2
Rash	2
Urinary abnormalities	2
* Placebo rates not available in package labeling.	
Physicians' Desk Reference. 57th ed. Montvale, NJ: Medical Economics Company, Inc; 2003:2236-2240.	

cally mediated and is not mediated by dosing levels. Risk factors associated with the development of agranulocytosis are:

- Increasing age
- Female gender
- Coadministration with other drugs causing hematologic complications
- Ashkenazi Jewish descent
- African American race.

The period of greatest risk for developing agranulocytosis is within the first 6 months after initiation of therapy. This is the rationale behind the mandate of the Food and Drug Administration (FDA) for weekly blood monitoring for the first 6 months. Thereafter, the frequency of monitoring is mandated to be every other week.

The clinical presenting symptoms of early stages of agranulocytosis include:

- Lethargy
- Weakness
- Fever
- Sore throat.

If the WBC count falls to <3000/mm^3 or the absolute neutrophil count (ANC) to <1500/mm^3, therapy with clozapine should be interrupted immediately. In a patient with a drop in WBC count to <2000/mm^3 or an ANC <1000/mm^3, clozapine should be discontinued and not be reinstated in the future.

Sedation

Drowsiness/sedation, as shown in Table 3.4, is the most frequently occurring side effect of clozapine therapy. It is usually transient and mild in the initial stages of therapy. Sedation is caused primarily by clozapine's antagonism of histamine (H)$_1$ receptors. Precautions to take in order to minimize clozapine-associated sedation include:

- Use of a minimal drug dose
- Bedtime drug administration
- Avoidance of other central nervous system (CNS) depressants.

Hypersalivation

Although salivation is reported in package labeling to occur in about one third of patients treated with clozapine, the reported incidence varies from 0% to 80%. Although the mechanism of hypersalivation is unknown, one explanation is that clozapine may act as an agonist at the muscarinic (M)$_4$ receptor leading to cholinergic activity and excess salivation. Nonetheless, subjective complaints of hypersalivation in clozapine-treated patients may not correlate with measured salivary flow rates. There is little systematic research on treatments for hypersalivation. Its severity often decreases over time during clozapine treatment. A few treatments have been found to be effective, but do not work in all instances (Table 3.5). These medications should only be used if behavioral programs (ie, initiating chewing gum) are not effective. It is not advisable to treat nocturnal salivation medically.

TABLE 3.5 — RECOMMENDED TREATMENTS OF HYPERSALIVATION

- Sugar-free gum
- Clonidine
- Low-dose benztropine, biperiden, or other anticholinergic agent
- Low-dose benztropine + terazosin combination

Cardiovascular and Respiratory Effects

Tachycardia is a relatively common side effect of clozapine treatment, occurring in about 25% of patients. Tachycardia may be related to rebound effects from related hypotension as well as clozapine-associated anticholinergic properties and its elevation of plasma norepinephrine. Tachycardia is usually transient but may require treatment with a peripheral β-blocking agent. Rarely, the tachycardia can be related to a type of rapid ventricular tachycardia known as torsades de pointes.

Orthostatic hypotension is often self-limiting and occurs transiently during clozapine initiation and titration. Orthostasis may occur with or without syncope; about 6% of patients will experience fainting. Dihydroergotamine has been used to alleviate orthostatic hypotension; however, there have been rare reports of respiratory arrest and cardiac arrest with the combination. Education about hypotension and advising the patient to rise slowly from a sitting or supine position are important and should be the mainstay of treatment during titration of the drug.

There are case reports of clozapine-associated cardiomyopathy and cardiorespiratory arrest. A black-box warning for myocarditis was recently added to package labeling. These reports have included patients with and without cardiac histories. Most of these cases involved coadministration of other agents (ie, benzodiazepines), further complicating interpretation of any causal relationship between clozapine and cardiorespiratory complications. Coadministration of benzodiazepines during initiation of clozapine should be avoided, if possible.

Seizures

The risk of seizure is dose-related in patients taking clozapine. The risk of seizure occurrence is 1% to 2% at doses <300 mg/day, similar to traditional antipsychotics. The risk of seizure is 3% to 4% at 300 to 600 mg/day doses and is 5% at doses >600 mg/day. Possible risk factors include:

- Rapid dose titration
- Previous history of neurologic abnormalities or preexisting seizure disorder
- Concomitant use of epileptogenic drugs.

Dosing >600 mg/day may warrant a baseline electroencephalogram (EEG). Types of seizures that may occur usually include:

- Tonic-clonic
- Complex partial
- Simple partial.

These seizures are usually preceded by myoclonic jerking. Decreasing the clozapine dose or adding an anticonvulsant, such as valproate or phenytoin, is effective treatment for preventing future seizure activity. Patients who are experiencing myoclonus should be monitored closely and possibly treated with an anticonvulsant to avoid a tonic-clonic seizure.

Weight Gain

Weight gain is a side effect associated with most antipsychotics. Clozapine, however, is associated with greater weight gain than most of the antipsychotic agents available. An average weight gain after 10 weeks of treatment is about 4.5 kg (9.9 lb). After 12 weeks of treatment, over two thirds of patients on clozapine will gain about 4 to 6 kg (8.8 to 13.2 lb), and 20% of patients will gain >10% of their baseline body weight. There has been no direct correlation between dosing and amount of weight gain. Nutrition counseling and exercise are the two most important recommendations that can be made to help reduce the amount of weight gain with this medication (see Chapter 7, *Metabolic Effects of Antipsychotic Drugs*).

Urinary Incontinence

Urinary incontinence occurs in about 1% of patients taking clozapine but is thought to be underreported because of the embarrassing nature of the adverse effect. Although the mechanism of urinary incontinence is not known, it is generally believed to occur due to the adrenergic antagonism of clozapine. This may lead to urinary incontinence through a mechanism leading to deceased internal bladder sphincter tone. Ephedrine, an α-adrenergic agonist, has been found to be effective in preventing urinary incontinence, as has desmopressin.

Olanzapine

■ History and Mechanism of Action

Olanzapine has a pharmacologic profile of activity similar to that of clozapine. In preclinical studies, olanzapine demonstrated a range of receptor affinities distinct from those of conventional antipsychotics and generally comparable to those of clozapine. However, in clinical trials, olanzapine has not been found to be as efficacious for treatment-resistant schizophrenia as is clozapine (see Chapter 11, *Treatment-Resistant Schizophrenia*). Olanzapine has greater affinity for 5-HT_{2A} than for D_2 receptors. In addition, the compound has affinity at the binding sites of D_4, D_3, 5-HT$_3$, 5-HT$_6$, H_1, α_1-adrenergic receptors, and M_{1-5} receptors.

■ Efficacy

Both American and international multicenter studies comparing olanzapine with haloperidol have found that olanzapine is effective in doses of 5.5 mg/day to 20 mg/day. Efficacy with respect to positive symptoms is equivalent to that of haloperidol. Olanzapine's efficacy regarding negative symptoms has been found to be equivalent or superior to that of haloperidol. The clinical trials that brought olanzapine to market compared a low (mean 6.6 mg/day), moderate (11.6 mg/day), and high dose (16.3 mg/day) of olanzapine. There were no significant differences in efficacy among dosage groups. However, the highest dose range appeared to offer the greatest benefit for both positive and negative symptoms compared with haloperidol.

■ Dosing

The recommended dosing for olanzapine is a once-daily dose beginning with 5 mg to 10 mg daily and reaching a target dose of 10 mg/day within several days. Dose increments/decrements are recommended to be 5 mg/day with a maximum dose of 15 to 20 mg/day. Since its introduction, the recommended dose of 10 mg/day has gravitated upward. The mean dose being utilized currently in the United States is around 18 mg/day. A few studies and reports on the use of olanzapine at doses of up to 50 mg/day are available. Greater efficacy at higher doses has not been demonstrated in controlled studies. Such doses should be used with caution.

■ Pharmacokinetics

Olanzapine is well absorbed following oral administration and can be given without regard to meals. The plasma protein binding of olanzapine is approximately 93%. Olanzapine is extensively metabolized in the liver to a number of inactive metabolites. The primary processes of metabolism are glucuronidation and demethylation by CYP450 1A2 (see Chapter 13, *Drug Interactions With Antipsychotic Drugs*). There is little metabolism of olanzapine occurring by the CYP450 2D6 pathway. The elimination half-life is approximately 31 hours; thus patients can be dosed once daily. Plasma drug levels have not been found to correlate with response, although there has been little work done in that area. The mean plasma concentration in males is approximately 35 ng/mL and 70 ng/mL in females after 8 weeks of treatment at 25-mg/day doses. Differences in plasma concentrations may be due to a slower metabolism or larger volume of distribution in women.

■ Adverse Effects

Table 3.6 lists spontaneously reported adverse effects as seen in clinical trials. Data on EPS can be found in Chapter 4, *Comparative Data Among Second-Generation Antipsychotic Drugs*.

Cardiovascular

Hypotension is reported to occur in 5% to 7% of patients taking olanzapine. Tachycardia occurs in approximately 4% of patients. Syncope was reported to occur in 0.6% of olanzapine-treated patients in phase II and III studies. The risk of orthostatic hypotension usually occurs within the initial dosing period and may be minimized by initiating therapy with a 5-mg/day dose. A more gradual titration to the target dose should be considered if hypotension occurs. Olanzapine should be used with caution in patients with known cardiovascular disease.

TABLE 3.6 — ADVERSE EFFECTS OF OLANZAPINE COMPARED WITH PLACEBO

Side Effect	Olanzapine (%)	Placebo (%)
Somnolence	29	13
Insomnia	12	11
Accidental injury	12	8
Dizziness	11	4
Asthenia	10	9
Constipation	9	4
Dry mouth	9	5
Dyspepsia	7	5
Rhinitis	7	6
Abnormal gait	6	1
Cough increased	6	3
Fever	6	2
Back pain	5	2
Ecchymosis	5	3
Extremity pain (other than joint)	5	3
Joint pain	5	3
Weight gain	5	3
Pharyngitis	4	3
Tremor	4	3
Vomiting	4	3
Akathisia	3	2
Amblyopia	3	2
Chest pain	3	1
Hypertonia	3	2
Increased appetite	3	2

Continued

Peripheral edema	3	1
Postural hypotension	3	1
Tachycardia	3	1
Articulation impairment	2	1
Hypertension	2	1
Urinary incontinence	2	1
Urinary tract infection	2	1

Physicians' Desk Reference. 57th ed. Montvale, NJ: Medical Economics Company, Inc; 2003:1877-1882.

Transaminase Elevations

In placebo-controlled studies, clinically significant alanine aminotransferase (ALT/SGPT) elevations of ≥3 times the upper limit of the normal range were observed in 2% of patients taking olanzapine. Also, during premarketing studies, the incidence of ALT elevations was 2%, but they were not associated with jaundice or other symptoms attributable to liver impairment. Transient increases may be seen but usually normalize with olanzapine continuation. One report of a patient with hepatitis C found persistent enzyme elevations for 4 months following discontinuation of olanzapine.

Weight Gain

Olanzapine, due to its propensity to block 5-HT_{2c} and H_1 receptors, may cause significant weight gain. In long-term trials (>1 year), weight gain ranged from 3.46 to 12.06 kg (7.6 to 26.6 lb). Thirty percent to 40% of patients can be expected to gain >7% of their body weight during olanzapine treatment. There is some evidence that weight gain with olanzapine may be related to dose, with larger gains occurring at higher doses. Many reports have found elevated lipids and fasting blood glucose levels occurring during olanzapine treatment. This is usually seen in people who have gained weight but has been reported in some patients in whom no weight gain has occurred (see Chapter 7, *Metabolic Effects of Antipsychotic Drugs*).

Quetiapine

■ **History and Mechanism of Action**

Structurally, quetiapine is related to clozapine and olanzapine. Quetiapine has high affinity for 5-HT_{2A} receptors and lower affinity for D_1 and D_2 receptors. This agent has some affinity for α_1 and α_2 receptors and H_1 receptors and very little for muscarinic receptors.

■ **Efficacy**

The efficacy of quetiapine for the treatment of psychosis was established in three short-term controlled trials. One trial evaluated five fixed doses (75 mg/day, 150 mg/day, 300 mg/day, 600 mg/day, and 750 mg/day) vs placebo. The maximum efficacy was found to occur at 300 mg/day. Another fixed-dose trial evaluated 50 mg/day vs 450 mg/day and found the higher dose to be superior. Additionally, quetiapine was tested in a flexible-dose study (<250 mg/day vs 250 to 750 mg/day). The mean dose was 360 mg/day in the high-dose group and 209 mg/day in the low-dose group. The greatest efficacy for positive symptoms occurred at doses >250 mg/day. In contrast to the other SGADs, quetiapine has not been shown to be superior to haloperidol in any symptom dimension, such as positive or negative symptoms.

■ **Dosing**

The dosing recommendations for quetiapine are initiation at a 25-mg dose twice daily, with increases by increments of 25 to 50 mg bid or tid on the second and third days, as tolerated, to a target dose range of 300 to 400 mg/day by the fourth day, given two or three times daily. Additional dosage adjustments of 25 to 50 mg bid should generally occur at intervals of not less that 2 days. The dose range for efficacy was found in trials to be 150 to 750 mg/day. Doses in the upper end of the recommended range appear to be most effective. Once daily dosing may be possible in stabilized patients.

■ Pharmacokinetics

Quetiapine is rapidly absorbed after oral administration. The bioavailability is marginally increased by administration with food. This agent is 83% bound to plasma proteins and is extensively metabolized by the liver. The enzyme involved with metabolism is the CYP450 3A4 and the two major metabolites are pharmacologically inactive. The elimination half-life is approximately 6 hours; thus quetiapine should be administered 2 to 4 times daily. To date, there are no good data on plasma concentrations and clinical response.

■ Adverse Effects

The spontaneously reported adverse effects from landmark clinical trials are listed in Table 3.7. Data on EPS can be found in Chapter 4, *Comparative Data Among Second-Generation Antipsychotic Drugs*.

Hypothyroidism

In clinical trials, a dose-related decrease in total and free thyroxine (T_4) of approximately 20% was seen in a few patients in the initial 2 to 4 weeks of treatment and maintained during chronic therapy. Generally, these changes were of no clinical significance and thyroid-stimulating hormone (TSH) was unchanged in most patients. Others have reported that

TABLE 3.7 — ADVERSE EFFECTS OF QUETIAPINE COMPARED WITH PLACEBO		
Side Effect	**Quetiapine** (%)	**Placebo** (%)
Headache	19	18
Somnolence	18	11
Dizziness	10	4
Constipation	9	5
Dry mouth	7	3
Postural hypotension	7	2
Tachycardia	7	5
Dyspepsia	6	2
Asthenia	4	3
Rash	4	3
Abdominal pain	3	1
Rhinitis	3	1
Back pain	2	1
Fever	2	1
Weight gain	2	0
Physicians' Desk Reference. 57th ed. Montvale, NJ: Medical Economics Company, Inc; 2003:681-685.		

<5% of patients experienced any changes. Approximately 0.4% (10/2386) of patients did experience TSH increases. Six of these patients with TSH increases needed thyroid-replacement therapy.

Cardiovascular

Quetiapine may cause orthostatic hypotension associated with dizziness, tachycardia, and in some patients, syncope. Syncope may occur in approximately 1% of patients treated, usually during the initial dose titration period. The risk of syncope and hypotension may be minimized by limiting the initial dosage to 25 mg bid. QT-wave prolongations and T-wave abnormalities have rarely been reported with quetiapine use.

Cataracts

Within manufacturer labeling, the warning for cataract development appears in bold ink, as required by the FDA. The warning states that the development of cataracts was observed in chronic dog studies and that examinations of the lens by slit lamp examination or other appropriately sensitive method to detect cataract formation is recommended at initiation and at 6-month intervals thereafter. There have been lens changes occurring in humans after long-term therapy, but a causal relationship has not been established. To date, there are no human reports of cataract formation during quetiapine therapy. The standard of care in the field in regard to this potential adverse effect is to ensure that there is an ophthalmoscopic examination performed within the previous 6 months prior to initiation, with follow-up examinations, if deemed necessary.

Transaminase Elevations

Asymptomatic transient and reversible elevations in plasma transaminases (primarily ALT) have been reported. Six percent of patients treated with quetiapine in clinical trials were found to have elevations of >3 times the upper limits of the normal reference range. Hepatic enzyme elevations generally occurred within the first 3 weeks of drug treatment and returned to pretreatment levels after discontinuation of quetiapine.

Weight Gain

Weight gain with quetiapine appears to be less than with clozapine and olanzapine and may be similar to that with risperidone treatment. In clinical trials, gains of 0.9 to 5.5 kg over 6 weeks were reported. In most studies, however, mean gains were around 2 kg over 6 weeks. Gain in weight appears to level off over time and does not appear to be dose related (see Chapter 7, *Metabolic Effects of Antipsychotic Drugs*).

Risperidone

■ History and Mechanism of Action

Risperidone, a benzisoxazole derivative, was first available in the United States in 1994. It has high binding affinity to both 5-HT_{2A} and D_2 receptors. Additionally, it binds to α_1 and α_2 receptors, with little blockade of cholinergic receptors.

■ Efficacy

Multicenter clinical trials that led to the FDA approval of risperidone found that its efficacy is at least equal to that of haloperidol and that it produces significantly fewer EPS. The US results of the United States–Canadian collaborative investigation were reported by Marder and Meibach in 1994. They reported that 6 mg/day of risperidone is superior to 20 mg/day of haloperidol. Fifty-seven percent of patients taking 6 mg/day of risperidone were found to have a 20% decrease in symptoms as measured by the Positive and Negative Syndrome Scale (PANSS). In comparison, only 30% receiving haloperidol and 22% receiving placebo also had this symptom reduction. EPS required that 47% of haloperidol-treated patients be treated with antiparkinsonian medication, while only 20% of those on risperidone 6 mg/day required treatment.

◼ Dosing

The initial package labeling for risperidone recommended that patients be titrated over 3 days to reach a dose of 6 mg (given as 3 mg twice daily). New labeling reflects more appropriate dosing of 4 to 8 mg once daily. Most trials demonstrate maximal efficacy at doses of ≤6 mg daily. Dosing should be initiated between 0.25 and 1 mg/day and titrated to between 2 and 4 mg/day in a few days. Some patients may require a slower titration. The safety of risperidone has not been evaluated above 16 mg/day. Patients should receive a trial of at least 4 to 6 weeks to maximize likelihood of response. EPS are dose related; therefore, patients treated with >6 mg/day will have a greater likelihood of EPS.

◼ Pharmacokinetics

Risperidone is well absorbed and the relative oral bioavailability from a tablet is 94%. Administration with food does not affect the rate or extent of absorption of risperidone; thus the drug can be given without regard to meals. Risperidone is extensively metabolized in the liver by CYP450 2D6 to a major active metabolite, 9-hydroxyrisperidone. This metabolite is approximately equal with respect to efficacy and receptor binding. Consequently, the clinical effect of the drug probably results from the combined effects of these compounds. The plasma protein binding of risperidone is 90% and the active metabolite is 70%. The half-life of risperidone is approximately 3 hours, while 9-hydroxyrisperidone has an elimination half-life of about 22 hours. This allows for once-daily dosing of risperidone. Plasma concentrations of either active compound have not yielded clinical information on blood levels and their relationships to response.

■ Adverse Effects

Spontaneously reported adverse effects from clinical trials are listed in Table 3.8. Data on EPS can be found in Chapter 4, *Comparative Data Among Second-Generation Antipsychotic Drugs*.

Cardiovascular

Because of risperidone's α-blocking activity, orthostatic hypotension may occur. Orthostasis may be associated with dizziness, tachycardia, and in some patients, syncope. Syncope occurs rarely, in approximately 0.2% of patients. Tachycardia has been reported to occur in approximately 3% of patients. Orthostatic hypotension is generally seen during the initial dose titration and is usually transient. Risperidone and its metabolite may, in rare cases, lengthen the QT interval. Clinical sequelae in known cases are rare; however, risperidone should be used with caution in patients with congenital QT prolongation, electrolyte imbalance, or concomitant use with other drugs that prolong the QT interval.

Prolactin-Related Adverse Effects

Dopamine-receptor antagonists increase prolactin production by inhibiting the action of dopamine on D_2 receptors in the pituitary. Risperidone causes a dose-dependent elevation of plasma prolactin levels of similar magnitude to those observed with haloperidol. Adverse effects related to prolactin elevation, such as amenorrhea, galactorrhea, gynecomastia, and ejaculatory and erectile dysfunction, appear to increase in a dose-related fashion. However, no direct correlation between plasma levels and adverse effects has been identified. At doses <6 mg/day, approximately 8% of women and men will report menstrual and/or sexual changes. At doses >6 mg/day, the number of patients experiencing prolactin-related problems may increase

TABLE 3.8 — ADVERSE EFFECTS OF RISPERIDONE COMPARED WITH PLACEBO

Side Effect	Risperidone (%)	Placebo (%)
Insomnia	26	19
Agitation	22	20
EPS	17	16
Headache	14	12
Anxiety	12	9
Rhinitis	10	4
Constipation	7	3
Nausea	6	3
Dyspepsia	5	4
Vomiting	5	4
Abdominal pain	4	0
Arthralgia	3	0
Tachycardia	3	0
Coughing	3	1
Somnolence	3	1
URI	3	1
Back pain	2	1
Chest pain	2	1
Dry skin	2	0
Fever	2	0
Pharyngitis	2	0
Toothache	2	0
Abnormal vision	2	1
Rash	2	1
Saliva increased	2	1
Sinusitis	2	1

Abbreviations: EPS, extrapyramidal symptoms; URI, upper respiratory infection.

Physicians' Desk Reference. 57th ed. Montvale, NJ: Medical Economics Company, Inc; 2003:1786-1790.

3

(see Chapter 4, *Comparative Data Among Second-Generation Antipsychotic Drugs*).

Weight Gain

Risperidone is associated with increased body weight in adults. In landmark trials, an average weight gain of 2.8 kg (6.2 lb) occurred after 8 weeks of treatment in adult patients randomized to receive 2 mg, 6 mg, 10 mg, or 16 mg of risperidone. No significant correlation has been found between weight gain and risperidone dose or plasma concentration. Eighteen percent of patients are expected to gain >7% of body weight during risperidone therapy. Risperidone treatment is associated with lower weight gain than olanzapine or clozapine treatment (see Chapter 7, *Metabolic Effects of Antipsychotic Drugs*).

Ziprasidone

■ History and Mechanism of Action

Ziprasidone was developed within a structure-activity investigation intended to find a compound that potently blocks D_2 receptors but binds with even greater affinity to central 5-HT_{2A} receptors. As a result, ziprasidone has a binding affinity ratio of 11:1 for 5-HT_{2A} and D_2. Ziprasidone also binds with relatively high affinity for 5-HT_{2C}, 5-HT_{1D}, α_1-adrenergic receptors, D_1, and D_3 receptors. Ziprasidone demonstrates potent partial agonist activism at the 5-HT_{1A} receptor.

■ Efficacy

The efficacy of ziprasidone was evaluated in five placebo-controlled trials. The first 4-week trial found ziprasidone 60 mg/day to be superior to placebo while this was not seen with the 20-mg/day dose. Another 4-week trial of 10, 40, and 80 mg/day did not find a difference vs placebo. A 6-week trial found both the 80- and 160-mg/day doses to be superior to placebo. Another 6-week trial also found no clear evidence of a dose response relationship, as the 40-, 120-, and 200-mg/day groups all were significantly greater than placebo for positive symptoms. Only the 200-mg/day dose was found to have efficacy for negative symptoms. One long-term study (52 weeks) with three fixed doses (40, 80, or 160 mg/day) found superiority to placebo at all doses in both time to relapse and rate of relapse. While haloperidol was compared with ziprasidone in one of the short-term trials, results of this arm of treatment has not been published. In a recent 28-week study, ziprasidone 80 mg was found to be similar to haloperidol 5 mg/day for the treatment of schizophrenia.

■ **Dosing**

The initial daily dosage of ziprasidone should be 20 mg bid with food. The maximum dosage, reached in approximately 2 to 3 days, is 80 mg bid. The safety and efficacy of dosages >100 mg bid have not been systematically studied. Clinical trials did not clearly delineate a superior dosage, although efficacy was demonstrated between 40 and 200 mg/day.

■ **Pharmacokinetics**

Absorption of ziprasidone is increased up to twofold in the presence of food, reaching an absolute bioavailability of approximately 60%. Ziprasidone is >99% bound to plasma proteins and has a mean volume of distribution of 1.5 L/kg. It is extensively metabolized by the CYP450 3A4 enzyme system (approximately one third) and oxidative metabolism by aldehyde oxidase (approximately two thirds). CYP450 1A2 may be involved to a minimal extent. The terminal half-life of ziprasidone is about 7 hours.

■ Adverse Effects

The adverse effects listed in Table 3.9 were spontaneously reported in short-term pivotal trials. Data on EPS and prolactin effects can be found in Chapter 4, *Comparative Data Among Second-Generation Antipsychotic Drugs.*

Cardiac Effects

Syncope and orthostatic hypotension occur infrequently and usually during the initial dose-titration period. Ziprasidone has the propensity to prolong the QTc interval. In placebo-controlled trials, ziprasidone increased the QTc interval compared with placebo by approximately 10 msec at 160 mg/day. Very few patients in clinical trials, however, had QTc intervals exceeding 500 msec, and no cases of torsades de pointes (TdP) have been reported, even in overdose situations. Ziprasidone should not be used with other drugs known to prolong the QTc interval such as:

- Quinidine
- Dofetilide
- Pimozide
- Sotalol
- Thioridazine
- Moxifloxacin
- Sparafloxacin.

This list is supplied by the manufacturer, but other drugs that have the potential for prolongation of the QTc can be found at www.torsades.org. There is a greater risk of QTc prolongation and TdP occurring in women. Other circumstances may place a patient at higher risk for occurrence of TdP and/or sudden death in association with ziprasidone, including bradycardia, hypokalemia, or hypomagnesemia, and the presence of congenital prolongation of the QT interval. Ziprasidone should be used with particular caution in patients with

TABLE 3.9 — ADVERSE EFFECTS OF ZIPRASIDONE COMPARED WITH PLACEBO

Side Effect	Ziprasidone (%)	Placebo (%)
Somnolence	14	7
Nausea	10	7
Constipation	9	8
Dizziness	8	6
Dyspepsia	8	7
Akathsia	8	7
Respiratory disorder	8	3
EPS	5	1
Diarrhea	5	4
Asthenia	5	3
Rhinitis	4	2
Accidental injury	4	2
Dry mouth	4	2
Dystonia	4	2
Rash	4	3
Abnormal vision	3	2
Cough increased	3	1
Hypertonia	3	2
Anorexia	2	1
Fungal dermatitis	2	1
Tachycardia	2	1

Abbreviation: EPS, extrapyramidal symptoms.

Physicians' Desk Reference. 57th ed. Montvale, NJ: Medical Economics Company, Inc; 2003:2601-2606.

known cardiovascular disease, cerebral vascular disease, or conditions that would predispose patients to hypotension. The safety of ziprasidone has been demonstrated in short-term trials with some metabolic inhibitors, but long-term studies, studies with other potent inhibitors such as erythromycin, and studies in chronic substance abusers have not been published.

Seizures

During clinical trials, seizures occurred in 0.4% of patients treated with ziprasidone. This drug should be used cautiously in patients with a history of seizures or with conditions that potentially lower the seizure threshold.

SUGGESTED READING

Arvanitis L, Miller B. Multiple fixed doses of "Seroquel" (quetiapine) in patients with acute exacerbation of schizophrenia: a comparison with haloperidol and placebo. The Seroquel Trial 13 Study Group. *Biol Psychiatry*. 1997;42:233-246.

Daniel DG, Zimbroff DL, Potkin SG, Reeves KR, Harrigan EP, Lakshminarayanan M. Ziprasidone 80 mg/day and 160 mg/day in the acute exacerbation of schizophrenia and schizoaffective disorders: a 6-week placebo-controlled trial. Ziprasidone Study Group. *Neuropsychopharmacology*. 1999;20:491-505.

Goff DC, Posever T, Herz L, et al. An exploratory haloperidol-controlled dose-finding study of ziprasidone in hospitalized patients with schizophrenia or schizoaffective disorder. *J Clin Psychopharmacol*. 1998;18:296-304.

Jordan S, Koprivica V, Chen R, Tottori K, Kikuchi T, Altar CA. The antipsychotic aripiprazole is a potent, partial agonist at the human 5-HT(1A) receptor. *Eur J Pharmacol*. 2002;441:137-140.

Kane JM, Carson WH, Saha AR, et al. Efficacy and safety of aripiprazole and haloperidol versus placebo in patients with schizophrenia and schizoaffective disorder. *J Clin Psychiatry*. 2002;63:763-771.

Lawler CP, Prioleau C, Lewis MM, et al. Interactions of the novel antipsychotic aripiprazole (OPC-14597) with dopamine and serotonin receptor subtypes. *Neuropsychopharmacology*. 1999;20: 612-627.

Marder SR, Meibach RC. Risperidone in the treatment of schizophrenia. *Am J Psychiatry*. 1994;151:825-835.

Matsubayashi H, Amano T, Sasa M. Inhibition by aripiprazole of dopaminergic inputs to striatal neurons from substantia nigra. *Psychopharmacology*. 1999;146:139-143.

Moore NA, Calligaro DO, Wong DT, et al. The pharmacology of olanzapine and other new antipsychotic agents. *Curr Opin Invest Drugs*. 1993;2:281-293.

Purdon SE. Cognitive improvement in schizophrenia with novel antipsychotic medications. *Schizophr Res*. 1999;35(suppl): S51-S60.

Stahl SM. Dopamine system stabilizers, aripiprazole, and the next generation of antipsychotics, part 1, "Goldilocks" actions at dopamine receptors. *J Clin Psychiatry*. 2001;62:841-842.

3

4

Comparative Data Among Second-Generation Antipsychotic Drugss

While much information about each second-generation antipsychotic drug (SGAD) is available, deciding among agents with regard to both efficacy and side effects is not as easily discernable. Very few large-scale trials that compare SGADs in a head-to-head fashion are available. This chapter will provide data available from direct-comparison trials of SGADs as well as combine existing data in a comparative fashion.

Receptor-Binding Profiles

Side effects of medication, as well as the efficacy of the antipsychotic drug, are largely explained by the receptor that the antipsychotic is blocking/stimulating. For example, sedation is related to high affinity for H_1 receptors. It was once believed that a higher ratio of 5-HT_{2A} to D_2 receptor blockade was needed for antipsychotic efficacy. This theory is not supported by the receptor affinity ratio of quetiapine and aripiprazole. Furthermore, aripiprazole functions as a partial agonist at the D_2 receptor, a unique pharmacologic mechanism in the SGAD class. Receptor affinities for SGADs are listed in Table 4.1.

Efficacy

Few data exist in regard to efficacy by direct head-to-head comparison studies between the SGADs. A meta-analysis is available on published trials comparing olanzapine, risperidone, and quetiapine with pla-

TABLE 4.1 — RECEPTOR AFFINITIES FOR SECOND-GENERATION ANTIPSYCHOTIC DRUGS

SGAD	Receptor Affinities									
	D_1	D_2	D_3	D_4	$5\text{-}HT_{1A}$	$5\text{-}HT_{2A}$	$5\text{-}HT_{2C}$	α_1	H_1	M_1
Aripiprazole*	265	0.34†	0.8	44	1.7	3.4	15	57	61	>1000
Clozapine	85	126	473	35	875	16	16	7	6	1.9
Olanzapine	31	11	49	27	>10,000	4	23	19	7	1.9
Quetiapine	455	160	340	1600	2800	295	1500	7	11	120
Risperidone	430	4	10	9	210	0.5	25	0.7	20	>10,000
Ziprasidone	525	5	7	32	3	0.4	1	11	50	>1000
Haloperidol‡	210	0.7	2	3	1100	45	>10,000	6	440	>1500

Abbreviations: D, dopamine; 5-HT, serotonin; H, histamine; M, muscarinic; SGAD, second-generation antipsychotic drug.

* In human cells that contain cloned receptors.

† Partial agonist activity at D_2 receptors; all others are D_2 antagonists.

‡ Conventional antipsychotic drug.

Arnt J, Skarsfeldt T. *Neuropsychopharmacology.* 1998;18:63-101; and Daniel DG, et al. *Neuropsychopharmacology.* 1999;20:491-505. Data on file for aripiprazole: Otsuka America Pharmaceutical, Inc., Rockville, Md.

cebo or haloperidol. All drugs were found to be more efficacious than placebo, while risperidone and olanzapine were more effective than haloperidol for global psychopathology and negative symptoms. Risperidone, olanzapine, and quetiapine were better than haloperidol with regard to extrapyramidal symptoms (EPS). Other data suggest that risperidone may be more effective for positive symptoms compared with haloperidol and olanzapine, but this has not been found for the other SGADs, excluding clozapine (Table 4.2).

Six large, comparative trials of the SGADs have been completed (Table 4.3). Overall, the studies determined that efficacy was similar overall in most domains. Large-scale, investigator-initiated, comparative trials are needed to clarify variances. There are important differences between these medications concerning pharmacokinetics, cost, and adverse effects.

TABLE 4.2 — EFFICACY OF SECOND-GENERATION ANTIPSYCHOTIC DRUGS COMPARED WITH HALOPERIDOL

Drug	Symptoms		
	Global	Positive	Negative
Aripiprazole	=	=	+
Olanzapine	+	=	+
Quetiapine	=	=	=
Risperidone	+	+	+
Ziprasidone	=	=	=
Key: +, superior; =, no difference.			

TABLE 4.3 — LARGE COMPARATIVE TRIALS OF SECOND-GENERATION ANTIPSYCHOTIC DRUGS		
Drug Comparison	Patient Population	Results
Risperidone vs olanzapine*	n = 339	Olanzapine > risperidone for negative and affective symptoms
Risperidone vs olanzapine*	n = 377	Risperidone > olanzapine for positive and affective symptoms
Risperidone vs quetiapine[†]	n = 216 (schizophrenia subset)	Comparable efficacy
Risperidone vs ziprasidone[‡]	n = 269	Comparable efficacy
Ziprasidone vs olanzapine[‡]	n = 296	Comparable efficacy
Risperidone vs aripiprazole[‡§]	n = 404	Comparable efficacy

* Published trials: Tran PV, et al. *J Clin Psychopharmacol.* 1997;17:407-418; and Conley RR, Mahmoud R. *Am J Psychiatry.* 2001;158:765-774.
† Larger sample with all diagnoses published; not schizophrenia subset.
‡ Data not yet published.
§ This study was not a head-to-head comparison of risperidone and aripiprazole but a comparison of risperidone and aripiprazole with placebo.

Adverse Effects

In clinical trials, rates of adverse effects with placebo are often relatively high. One measure of separating side effect rates that are high compared with those with placebo is to look at all adverse effects that occurred in ≥5% of patients and those that occurred at twice the rate of placebo. A comparison of these side effects among SGADs as shown in their package inserts appears in Table 4.4. Comparative data on tolerability and safety of SGADs are presented. Data for weight gain are located in Chapter 7, *Metabolic Effects of Antipsychotic Drugs*.

The incidence of sedation, anticholinergic effects, and orthostatic hypotension are to a great extent related to the antagonism at H_1, M_1, and alpha-1 (α_1) receptors, respectively (Table 4.5).

■ Extrapyramidal Side Effects

It is well accepted that *in vitro* binding affinity of antipsychotics to the D_2 receptors predicts the likelihood of causing EPS. This relationship has been supported by *in vivo* radioligand binding studies with positron emission tomography. Blockade of $5\text{-}HT_{2A}$ receptors may mitigate against the EPS of these drugs. The comparative D_2 receptor blockades are shown in Figure 4.1

Much of the clinical advantage favoring SGADs comes from the fact that there is a wider separation between doses that cause EPS compared with effective doses of these drugs vs conventional antipsychotics (Figure 4.2). This property may lead to a better quality of life and greater adherence in people who are prescribed the SGADs.

Clinically, the rates of EPS are comparable to the *in vitro* binding. Clozapine is associated with little or no EPS, and quetiapine and aripiprazole have been found to have no greater rates of EPS than placebo.

TABLE 4.4 — COMPARISON OF SIDE EFFECTS AMONG SECOND-GENERATION ANTIPSYCHOTIC DRUGS THAT OCCURRED IN ≥5% OF PATIENTS AND AT TWICE THE RATE OF PLACEBO

Aripiprazole*	Clozapine	Olanzapine	Quetiapine	Risperidone	Ziprasidone	Haloperidol†
None	Sedation Vertigo Headache Sweating Visual disturbances Tachycardia Hypotension Syncope Constipation Nausea Fever	Postural hypotension Constipation Weight gain Dizziness Personality disorder Akathisia	Dizziness Postural hypotension Dry mouth Dyspepsia	Anxiety Sedation EPS Dizziness Constipation Nausea Dyspepsia Rhinitis Rash Tachycardia	Sedation EPS Respiratory disorder	EPS Anxiety Sedation Tachycardia Constipation Hypotension

Abbreviation: EPS, extrapyramidal symptoms.

* Adverse events that occurred in ≥2% of patients treated with aripiprazole and greater than the incidence in patients treated with placebo include headache, anxiety, insomnia, nausea, vomiting, somnolence, light-headedness, constipation, akathisia, rash, rhinitis, asthenia, coughing, tremor, blurred vision, and fever.

† Conventional antipsychotic drug.

TABLE 4.5 — ADVERSE EFFECTS OF SECOND-GENERATION ANTIPSYCHOTIC DRUGS

Drug	Sedation	Anticholinergic Effects	Orthostatic Hypotension
Aripiprazole	+	0/+	0/+
Clozapine	+++	+++	+++
Olanzapine	++	++	++
Quetiapine	++	0	+
Risperidone	+	0/+	+
Ziprasidone	+	0/+	++

Key: 0 (absent), + (minimal), ++ (mild), +++ (moderate).

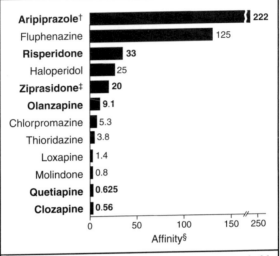

FIGURE 4.1 — DOPAMINE-2 RECEPTOR AFFINITY OF ANTIPSYCHOTIC DRUGS*

Drug	Affinity
Aripiprazole[†]	222
Fluphenazine	125
Risperidone	33
Haloperidol	25
Ziprasidone[‡]	20
Olanzapine	9.1
Chlorpromazine	5.3
Thioridazine	3.8
Loxapine	1.4
Molindone	0.8
Quetiapine	0.625
Clozapine	0.56

Second-generation antipsychotic drug names are bold-faced.

* Affinity data were compiled from: Richelson E, Nelson A. *Eur J Pharmacol.* 1984;103:197-204; Moore NA, et al. *Curr Opin Invest Drugs.* 1993;2:281-293; Hyttel J, et al. *Clin Neuropharmacol.* 1992;15:267a-268a.
† Data on file for aripiprazole: Otsuka America Pharmaceutical, Inc., Rockville, Md. Partial D_2 agonist activity.
‡ Adapted from: Daniel DG, et al. *Neuropsychopharmacology.* 1999;20:491-505.
§ $10^{-7} \times 1/K_d$ where K_d = equilibrium dissociation in molarity.

Adapted from: Richelson E. *J Clin Psychiatry.* 1996:57(suppl 11):4-11.

Olanzapine and risperidone both cause EPS less often than do conventional antipsychotics but in a dose-related fashion. Ziprasidone also has a very low incidence of EPS, only slightly higher than placebo rates. Figure 4.3 shows the incidence of EPS in trials of all

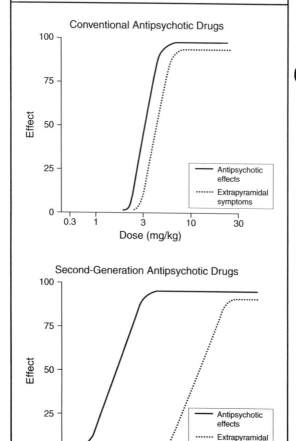

FIGURE 4.2 — EXTRAPYRAMIDAL SYMPTOM CURVES FOR CONVENTIONAL AND SECOND-GENERATION ANTIPSYCHOTIC DRUGS

Conventional Antipsychotic Drugs

Effect

Dose (mg/kg)

Antipsychotic effects

Extrapyramidal symptoms

Second-Generation Antipsychotic Drugs

Effect

Dose (mg/kg)

Antipsychotic effects

Extrapyramidal symptoms

Casey DE. *Int Clin Psychopharmacol*. 1995;10(suppl 3):105-114.

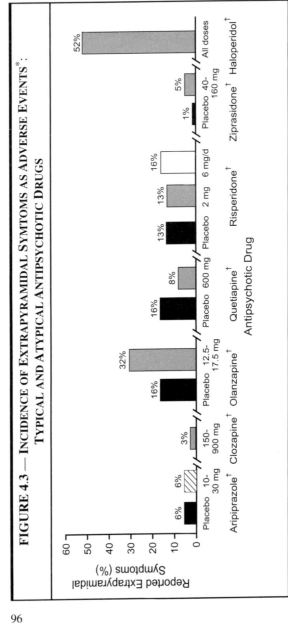

FIGURE 4.3 — INCIDENCE OF EXTRAPYRAMIDAL SYMTOMS AS ADVERSE EVENTS[*]: TYPICAL AND ATYPICAL ANTIPSYCHOTIC DRUGS

* In short-term, placebo-controlled trials.

† Percentages of extrapyramidal symptoms are derived from US labeling and include the following terminology: acute dystonia, parkinsonism, akathisia, tardive dyskinesia, dystonic events, dyskinetic events, akinesia, rigiditiy, extrapyramidal syndrome, hypertonia, neck rigidity, and tremor.

Data from: *Physicians' Desk Reference.* 56th ed. Medical Economics Company, Inc; Montvale, NJ. 2002. Data on file for aripiprazole: Otsuka America Pharmaceutical, Inc., Rockville, Md.

4

SGADs. Tardive dyskinesia with all of the SGADs appears to occur at an incidence of <2%, but few long-term follow-up studies are currently available.

■ Prolactin-Related Adverse Effects/ Sexual Dysfunction

Sexual functioning has received little attention or recognition as being an important aspect of patient care for those suffering from severe mental disorders such as schizophrenia. A recent survey identified that the area of personal relationships is one of the treatment areas with the most unmet needs as noted by people with schizophrenia. It is likely that a better focus on sexuality and preventing sexual dysfunction in schizophrenia would be a major benefit for improving treatment.

Sexual dysfunction during antipsychotic therapy can be attributed to several mechanisms (Table 4.6). In men, it appears that the most commonly reported sexual side effects associated with traditional antipsychotics are erection and ejaculation disturbances (30% to 60%). Difficulty achieving and maintaining erection is a common complaint as is delayed or inhibited ejaculation and retrograde and spontaneous

---

TABLE 4.6 — MECHANISMS OF SEXUAL DYSFUNCTION DURING ANTIPSYCHOTIC DRUG THERAPY

- Sedation
- Weight gain
- Extrapyramidal side effects
- Tardive dyskinesia
- Serotonin antagonism
- Cholinergic antagonism
- α-Adrenergic blockade
- Calcium channel blockade
- Dopamine antagonism (prolactin elevations)

---

ejaculation. Diminished libido and decreased orgasm quality are also commonly reported in men. Priapism, a sustained painful erection that can result in permanent impotence, has also been reported. Women report decreased libido and orgasmic dysfunction, including difficulty achieving orgasm, changes in the quality of orgasm, and anorgasmia. Fifty to ninety percent of women experience menstrual irregularities with conventional antipsychotic treatment. Women may also experience dyspareunia secondary to vaginal atrophy and dryness. Galactorrhea in both sexes and gynecomastia in males are also known to occur and may be more pronounced in younger patients.

Only a handful of articles, other than case reports, exist that discuss sexual functioning with the use of SGADs. The incidence of sexual disturbances with the use of SGADs is low as reported in the patient monographs. However, spontaneous reports may be underreported in all SGAD trials. Clozapine has a low propensity to block dopamine in the tuberinfundibular pathway and has a negligible effect on plasma prolactin levels. Sexual function during clozapine treatment has been comparatively better than during treatment with conventional antipsychotics and possibly risperidone. Case reports of priapism and impotence with clozapine have been reported and are likely related to α-adrenergic and muscarinic blockade as opposed to being related to hyperprolactinemia. Amenorrhea, galactorrhea, and gynecomastia are rare during clozapine treatment.

Of all the SGADs, risperidone has the highest propensity to elevate plasma prolactin levels and does so in a dose-related fashion. Mean prolactin levels at doses of 3 mg are about 27 ng/mL, significantly higher than olanzapine or clozapine. Studies in which patients have been actively questioned have produced higher reported rates as menstrual changes were reported to occur in 24% of patients treated with risperidone and

20% with olanzapine. Several case reports in the literature describe sexual dysfunction during risperidone treatment. For male patients, reports describe gynecomastia, galactorrhea, ejaculatory difficulties, and priapism occurring during risperidone treatment. In women, menstrual irregularities are the most commonly reported and have occurred at doses as low as 1 mg/day. Amenorrhea and galactorrhea are also reported to occur with fairly low doses of risperidone.

Olanzapine causes transient elevations in plasma prolactin levels. During treatment in adults, prolactin levels remain slightly elevated in about one third of patients. Elevation of prolactin appears to be a dose-related phenomenon. During 10- to 30-mg daily treatment with olanzapine, mean prolactin levels are approximately 17 ng/mL, which is higher than those in normals, drug-free patients, and clozapine-treated patients. Possibly because of its lower propensity to elevate prolactin, few case reports have been published with regard to sexual dysfunction and menstrual changes with use of this agent. No systematic studies, however, have been completed to specifically measure this side effect. At least seven case reports have discussed the occurrence of priapism with olanzapine treatment; this may be due to the alpha and muscarinic blockade of this medication. Comparative data, however, from one large clinical trial using routine doses of olanzapine and risperidone found rates of sexual dysfunction to be approximately 30% in males in both medication groups.

Quetiapine has negligible effects on the elevation of prolactin. In all of the large trials of quetiapine, prolactin levels were reported to decrease from baseline to end point during quetiapine treatment, and no differences were noted between quetiapine and placebo. In over 2,000 patients treated with quetiapine, menstrual changes occurred in <1% of patients. No cases of sexual dysfunction at standard doses have appeared in the literature to date.

Very few data are available pertaining to either plasma prolactin levels or sexual functioning with ziprasidone; it appears that slight elevations may occur with ziprasidone. In a double-blind study, prolactin levels were approximately 19 ng/mL and 60 ng/mL with ziprasidone and risperidone treatment, respectively, at the end of 52 weeks. Impotence, abnormal ejaculation, amenorrhea, galactorrhea, and anorgasmia occurred infrequently (<0.1%) in premarketing studies.

Prolactin levels while a patient is taking aripiprazole remain unaffected or decreased only slightly. Very few data on sexual dysfunction are available, and some studies have shown greater decreases in prolactin from baseline to end point as compared with placebo. Long-term studies have shown no emergence of prolactin elevations. Further study is needed; however, partial dopamine agonist activity may contribute to these findings.

Several treatment issues should be addressed when a patient complains of sexual disturbances (see Table 4.7). Initiating antipsychotics that have a lower propensity to elevate prolactin or cause sexual dysfunction should be considered in patients who are concerned about this issue or have a history of sexual dysfunction.

■ Effects on the QTc interval

The QT interval is the period extending from the beginning of depolarization (QRS complex) to the end of repolarization (T wave) of the ventricles. The QT interval is shorter with faster heart rates and longer with slower heart rates. Therefore, a correction for rate (the corrected QT or QTc) is applied to make the reporting of the interval more meaningful. QTc intervals are generally considered to be prolonged if they are

TABLE 4.7 — TREATMENT OPTIONS FOR SEXUAL DISTURBANCES

- Relationship counseling
- Rule out concomitant medications (anticholinergic and antidepressant medications)
- Rule out other secondary causes (weight gain and diabetes)
- Lowering dose
- Switching antipsychotics
- Pharmacologic intervention (last resort):
  – Sildenafil
  – Bethanechol
  – Cyproheptadine
  – Bromocriptine (should rarely be used due to exacerbation of illness)

>450 msec in males or 470 msec in females. In either gender, QTc prolongation >500 msec may place a patient at higher risk for torsades de pointes (TdP), a life-threatening condition. Recently, the effects of antipsychotic drugs on the QTc have received more attention. In a large study, it was reported that out of 20 classes of psychotropic medications studied, droperidol and thioridazine were the most likely to cause QTc prolongation. Most SGADs have some propensity to prolong the QTc, yet no cases of TdP have been reported even in overdose situations. The mean change from baseline in the QTc interval is shown in Figure 4.4.

Numerous factors have now been demonstrated to predispose patients to QTc prolongation. In addition to the role that medications play, major risk factors and possible contributing variables include:

- Metabolic abnormalities:
  – Hypokalemia
  – Hypomagnesemia
  – Hypothyroidism
  – Hypocalcemia

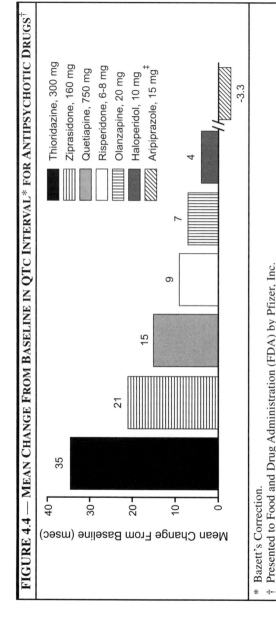

FIGURE 4.4 — MEAN CHANGE FROM BASELINE IN QTC INTERVAL* FOR ANTIPSYCHOTIC DRUGS[†]

Legend:
- Thioridazine, 300 mg
- Ziprasidone, 160 mg
- Quetiapine, 750 mg
- Risperidone, 6-8 mg
- Olanzapine, 20 mg
- Haloperidol, 10 mg
- Aripiprazole, 15 mg[‡]

Values (Mean Change From Baseline, msec):
35, 21, 15, 9, 7, 4, -3.3

Y-axis: Mean Change From Baseline (msec)

* Bazett's Correction.
† Presented to Food and Drug Administration (FDA) by Pfizer, Inc.
‡ Data on file for aripiprazole: Otsuka America Pharmaceutical, Inc., Rockville, Md.

103

- Female gender
- Hyperglycemia
- Alcoholism
- Bradycardia
- Cardiac disease:
  - Myocarditis
  - Heart failure
  - Myocardial ischemia
  - Myocardial infarction
- Rheumatic fever
- Mitral valve prolapse
- Low-energy diets
- Consumption of a large meal
- Obesity
- Parkinson's disease
- Liver disease
- Renal insufficiency
- Congenital long QT syndrome (LQTS) (1:5000)
- Jervell and Lange-Nielsen syndrome (autosomal recessive with deafness)
- Romano-Ward syndrome (autsomal dominant without deafness).

Only ziprasidone carries a warning of QTc prolongation in package labeling. It prolongs the QTc approximately 6 to 21 seconds longer than all other SGADs. Ziprasidone should not be used with other medications known to prolong the QTc.

SUGGESTED READING

Aizenberg D, Modai I, Landa A, Gil-Ad I, Weizman A. Comparison of sexual dysfunction in male schizophrenic patients maintained on treatment with classical antipsychotics versus clozapine. *J Clin Psychiatry.* 2001;62:541-544.

Andersson C, Chakos M, Mailman R, Lieberman J. Emerging roles for novel antipsychotic medications in the treatment of schizophrenia. *Psychiatr Clin North Am.* 1998;21:151-179.

Brown CS, Markowitz JS, Moore TR, Parker NG. Atypical antipsychotics: Part II: Adverse effects, drug interactions, and costs. *Ann Pharmacother.* 1999;33:210-217.

Casey DE. Motor and mental aspects of extrapyramidal syndromes. *Int Clin Psychopharmacol.* 1995;10(suppl 3):105-114.

Collaborative Working Group on Clinical Trial Evaluations. Measuring outcome in schizophrenia: differences among the atypical antipsychotics. *J Clin Psychiatry.* 1998;59(suppl 12):3-9.

Conley RR, Mahmoud R. A randomized double-blind study of risperidone and olanzapine in the treatment of schizophrenia or schizoaffective disorder. *Am J Psychiatry.* 2001;158:765-774.

Dickson RA, Glazer WM. Hyperprolactinemia and male sexual dysfunction. *J Clin Psychiatry.* 1999;60:125.

Fayek M, Kingsbury SJ, Zada J, Simpson GM. Cardiac effects of antipsychotic medications. *Psychiatr Serv.* 2001;52:607-609.

Leucht A, Pitschel-Walz G, Abraham D, Kissling W. Efficacy and extrapyramidal side-effects of the new antipsychotics olanzapine, quetiapine, risperidone, and sertindole compared to conventional antipsychotics and placebo. A meta-analysis of randomized controlled trials. *Schizophr Res.* 1999;35:51-68.

Marder SR, Meibach RC. Risperidone in the treatment of schizophrenia. *Am J Psychiatry.* 1994;151:825-835.

Moore NA, Calligaro DO, Wong DT, et al. The pharmacology of olanzapine and other new antipsychotic agents. *Curr Opin Invest Drugs.* 1993;2:281-293.

Purdon SE. Cognitive improvement in schizophrenia with novel antipsychotic medications. *Schizophr Res.* 1999;35(suppl): S51-S60.

Reilly JG, Ayis SA, Ferrier IN, Jones SJ, Thomas SH. QTc-interval abnormalities and psychotropic drug therapy in psychiatric patients. *Lancet.* 2000;355:1048-1052.

Remington G, Kapur S. D2 and 5-HT2 receptor effects of antipsychotics: bridging basic and clinical findings using PET. *J Clin Psychiatry.* 1999;60(suppl 10):15-19.

Richelson E. Preclinical pharmacology of neuroleptics: focus on new generation compounds. *J Clin Psychiatry.* 1996;57(suppl 11):4-11.

Richelson E, Nelson A. Antagonism by neuroleptics of neurotransmitter receptors of normal human brain *in vitro. Eur J Pharmacol.* 1984;103:197-204.

Tran PV, Hamilton SH, Kuntz AJ, et al. Double-blind comparison of olanzapine versus risperidone in the treatment of schizophrenia and other psychotic disorders. *J Clin Psychopharmacol.* 1997;17: 407-418.

Yap YG, Camm J. Risk of torsades de pointes with non-cardiac drugs. Doctors need to be aware that many drugs can cause qt prolongation. *Br Med J.* 2000;320:1158-1159.

5 Conventional Antipsychotic Drugs

History

Antipsychotic drugs have been in clinical use since the 1950s when chlorpromazine was synthesized in France. It was first used as a preanesthetic agent. Within 2 years of use, it was found to be effective in the treatment of psychotic patients. Many other similar medications followed in the next decade. These medications were commonly referred to as neuroleptics, which means "causing a neurologic disorder." This name came about due to the profound extrapyramidal symptoms (EPS) they produce. Many believed the induction of motor side effects was necessary, however, for efficacy of the medications.

Mechanism of Action and Structures

All of the conventional antipsychotic agents available are high-affinity dopamine $(D)_2$ receptor antagonists. Among the conventional compounds, although there are some differences in their affinities for D_1 and D_2 receptors, these differences do not appear to be clinically significant. These agents block 65% to 80% of D_2 receptors in the striatum during chronic treatment and block dopamine in the other three dopamine tracts as well.

Phenothiazines, the first chemical class of antipsychotic drugs developed, are tricyclic molecules. Three subtypes of phenothiazines are available:
- Aliphatics
- Piperidines
- Piperazines.

These subtypes differ chemically, depending on the substituent on a ring-nitrogen. The phenothiazines with aliphatic side chains tend to be low-potency compounds (ie, higher equivalent doses are needed to achieve therapeutic effectiveness). Piperidine substitutions have anticholinergic properties and a lower incidence of EPS. Piperazine agents are the most potent of the phenothiazines. Other than the phenothiazines, classes available are:

- Thioxanthenes
- Butyrophenones
- Diphenylbutylpiperidines
- Dihydroindolones
- Dibenzodiazepines (Figure 5.1).

Efficacy and Dosing

All conventional antipsychotics are equivalent in efficacy when used in equipotent doses (see Chapter 2, *Treatment of Schizophrenia*). Interindividual variation does occur between traditional antipsychotics such that a relatively responsive patient may not respond equally to each antipsychotic. Selection of medication should be based on the need to avoid certain side effects based on patient variables or concurrent medical or psychiatric disorders. There are no differences in efficacy between the low- and high-potency agents. Previous family history of response is also helpful in the selection of an agent. Traditional dosage equivalents (expressed in chlorpromazine [CPZ]-equivalent dosages) are the equipotent dosages of any of the traditional antipsychotics compared with 100 mg CPZ. The usual recommendation for initiation of therapy is 400 CPZ to 600 CPZ equivalents unless the patient's history indicates that this dose may result in unacceptable adverse effects. Maintenance therapy should provide a dose of 300 CPZ to 600 CPZ equivalents for maximum efficacy. In the 1970s and

1980s, large doses were utilized with the belief that larger daily doses were necessary in more severely symptomatic patients. Randomized controlled trials have found no difference in efficacy between recommended and high-dose therapies. Information on available dosage forms and dosing is provided in Tables 5.1 and 5.2.

Pharmacokinetics

Conventional antipsychotics are generally well absorbed through the gastrointestinal tract and undergo extensive first-pass hepatic metabolism. Food and antacids may decrease absorption. Liquid preparations are absorbed more rapidly and reliably than tablets and capsules. Antipsychotic drugs are generally highly protein bound (85% to 90%). These agents are highly lipophilic; thus they readily cross the blood-brain barrier and attain high concentrations in the brain. Given their high degree of protein and tissue binding, these drugs are not removed efficiently by dialysis. The elimination half-life of most of the conventional antipsychotics is 18 to 40 hours; therefore, most agents can be administered once daily, side effects permitting.

Most of the agents are metabolized in the liver to demethylated and hydroxylated forms. Several of the hydroxyl and desmethyl metabolites of the phenothiazines are active as dopamine antagonists. Chlorpromazine has an active metabolite, 7-hydroxychlorpromazine fluphenazine is metabolized to 7-hydroxyfluphenazine; and thioridazine is metabolized to mesoridazine. Haloperidol, perphenazine, and thioridazine are metabolized by the cytochrome P450 (CYP450) 2D6 isoenzyme (see Chapter 13, *Drug Interactions With Antipsychotic Drugs*). The measurement of plasma levels has not correlated well with response. Currently, haloperidol is the only agent on which some consistent data on plasma level to re-

FIGURE 5.1 — STRUCTURE OF CONVENTIONAL ANTIPSYCHOTIC DRUGS

Aliphatic Phenothiazine

Chlorpromazine

Piperazine Phenothiazines

Fluphenazine

Perphenazine

Trifluoperazine

Piperidine Phenothiazines

Mesoridazine

Thioridazine

Thioxanthene

Thiothixene

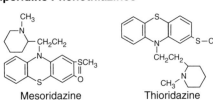

Butyrophenone

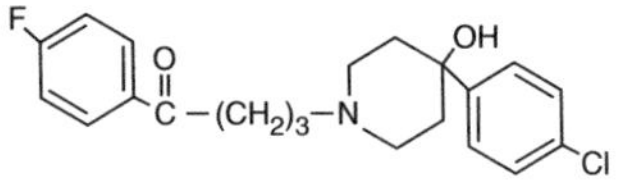

Haloperidol

Dibenzoxazepine

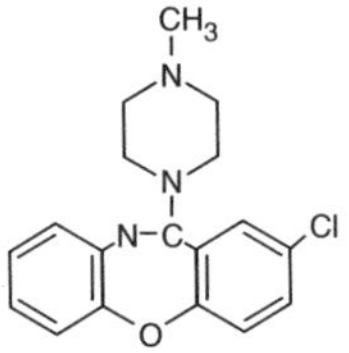

Loxapine

Dihydroindolone

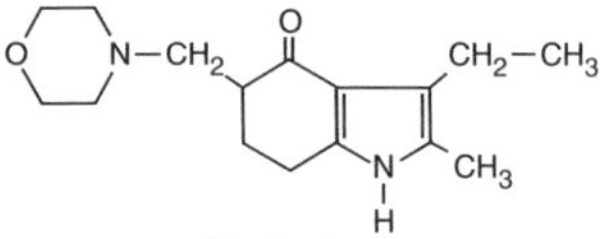

Molindone

Diphenylbutylpiperidine

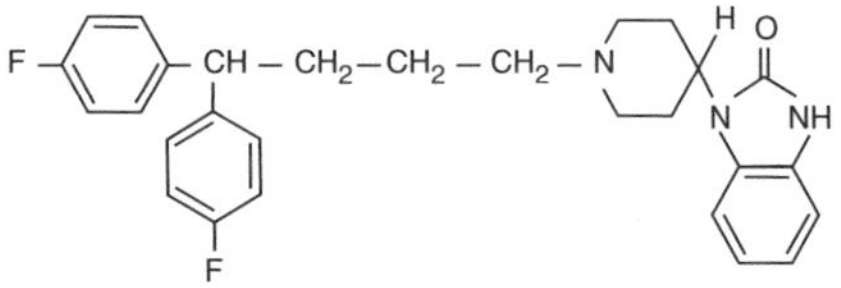

Pimozide

TABLE 5.1 — AVAILABLE PREPARATIONS OF CONVENTIONAL ANTIPSYCHOTIC DRUGS				
Drug	Tablets (mg)	Liquid (mg/mL)	Parenteral (mg/mL)	Other
Chlorpromazine	10, 25, 50, 100, 200	10/5, 30, 100	25	30-, 75-, 150-mg sustained-release capsules; 25-, 100-mg rectal suppositories
Fluphenazine	1, 2.5, 5, 10	2.5/5, 5	2.5	25 mg/mL decanoate; 25 mg/mL enanthate
Haloperidol	0.5, 1, 2, 5, 10, 20	2	5	50 mg/mL, 100 mg/mL decanoate (intramuscular only)
Loxapine	—	25	50 (intramuscular only)	5-, 10-, 25-, 50-mg capsules
Mesoridazine	10, 25, 50, 100	25	25	—
Molindone	5, 10, 25, 50, 100	20	—	—
Perphenazine	2, 4, 8, 16	16/5	5	—

Pimozide	2	—	—	—
Trifluoperazine	1, 2, 5, 10	10	2	—
Thioridazine	10, 15, 25, 50, 100, 150, 200	25/5, 100/5, 30, 100	—	—
Thiothixene	—	5	—	1-, 2-, 5-, 10-, 20-mg capsules

TABLE 5.2 — DOSING INFORMATION FOR CONVENTIONAL ANTIPSYCHOTIC DRUGS	
Drug	**Dosage Range** (mg/day)
Chlorpromazine	300 to 800
Fluphenazine	2 to 40
Haloperidol	5 to 30
Loxapine	25 to 100
Mesoridazine	150 to 500
Molindone	25 to 100
Perphenazine	8 to 64
Pimozide	1 to 10
Thioridazine	300 to 700
Thiothixene	5 to 40
Trifluoperazine	15 to 30

sponse are available. There is evidence that haloperidol levels >5 to 10 ng/mL may correspond with clinical antipsychotic effects.

Decanoates

Depot preparations of two antipsychotics (fluphenazine decanoate and enanthate, and haloperidol decanoate) are available in the United States. These are esterified antipsychotics formulated in sesame seed oil for deep intramuscular (IM) injection. Because these are long-acting preparations, patients should be exposed to the oral form of the drug prior to their first injection to minimize the possibility of long-acting side effects. With initial dosing, oral supplementation may temporarily be necessary. Care must be taken not to increase the depot preparation too rapidly because steady state is only reached after 4 to 5 dosing intervals (see Chapter 9, *Long-Acting Antipsychotic Drugs*).

Adverse Effects of Conventional Antipsychotic Drugs

Conventional antipsychotics cause a wide range of adverse events, affecting many organ systems. In general, the adverse effects of the low-potency agents are more non-neurologic in nature and the higher potency agents cause most adverse neurologic effects. Most, but not all, of the adverse effects seen with these agents can be categorized by the neurotransmitter system affected (Table 5.3).

TABLE 5.3 — ADVERSE EFFECTS ASSOCIATED WITH RECEPTOR ANTAGONISM	
Receptor	**Adverse Effect**
Histamine-1	Sedation, weight gain
Muscarinic	Urinary retention, dry mouth, blurred vision, constipation, sinus tachycardia, cognition and memory deficits
Alpha-1	Orthostatic hypotension, reflex tachycardia, miosis
Serotonin-2C	Weight gain
Dopamine-2	Extrapyramidal symptoms, hyperprolactinemia/sexual dysfunction

Sedation, anticholinergic effects, and cardiovascular effects are all dependent upon the potency of the antipsychotic. The lower-potency agents cause these adverse effects at a higher rate (Table 5.4).

TABLE 5.4 — ADVERSE EFFECTS OF CONVENTIONAL ANTIPSYCHOTIC DRUGS

Drug	Sedation	Anticholinergic Effect	Cardiovascular Effect
Chlorpromazine	++++	+++	++++
Fluphenazine	++	++	++
Haloperidol	+	+	+
Loxapine	+++	++	+++
Mesoridazine	+++	+++	+++
Molindone	+	++	++
Perphenazine	++	++	++
Thioridazine	++++	++++	++++
Thiothixene	++	++	++
Trifluoperazine	++	++	++

Key: + (very low), ++ (low), +++ (moderate), ++++ (high).

■ Sedation

Sedation is primarily a result of the blockade of histamine $(H)_1$ receptors. The low-potency agents are the most sedating of the conventional antipsychotics. Oversedation may decrease cognitive, perceptual, and motor dysfunction. Thus patients should be warned about driving or operating machinery when first treated with these agents. The entire dose may be given at bedtime to decrease daytime drowsiness. Tolerance to sedation usually develops after several weeks.

■ Cardiovascular Side Effects

The low-potency agents are more cardiotoxic than the high-potency drugs. Chlorpromazine and thioridazine, in particular, cause prolongation of the QT and PR intervals, blunting of T-waves, and depression of the ST segment. Thus the piperidine phenothiazines are the most lethal among the antipsychotics in overdose situations. Torsades de pointes has been reported with thioridazine, possibly due to its sulfoxide metabolite, which may cause sudden death. Nonetheless, most electrocardiogram (ECG) changes that occur when normal therapeutic doses are given to physically healthy patients are not usually clinically significant. In patients over 40 years of age, a pretreatment ECG is recommended.

Orthostatic (postural) hypotension, defined as a drop in systolic pressure >20 mm Hg, most frequently occurs with chlorpromazine and thioridazine. Reflex vasoconstriction when rising to a sitting or standing position is inhibited when α-adrenergic receptors are blocked. This appears to be caused by a combination of local vasodilatory effects and central inhibition of the vasomotor center, as well as sympatholysis leading to unopposed β-adrenergic effects. This side effect most frequently occurs when high doses are given via the IM route and during the first few days of oral treatment. Patients usually gain a tolerance to orthostasis within a few days. The primary danger of orthostasis is that patients may fall or faint and injure themselves. Elderly patients, diabetic patients, and those with preexisting cardiovascular disease may be most predisposed.

When beginning treatment with low-potency agents, the patient should be warned of the adverse effects and advised to rise from bed gradually, sit at first with their legs dangling, wait a minute, and sit or lie down if they feel faint. Additionally, the clinician should measure the patient's blood pressure (supine and standing, separated by several minutes) before and after the first several days of treatment. If hypotension continues to occur, the symptoms can usually be managed by having patients lie down with their feet higher than their head. Support hose may be of benefit. If orthostasis persists, switching to a higher-potency agent or a second-generation antipsychotic drug (SGAD) is warranted. Rarely would volume-expansion or vasopressor agents (eg, norepinephrine) be used.

■ **Anticholinergic Effects**

Chlorpromazine, thioridazine, mesoridazine, and trifluoperazine are the most potent anticholinergic agents among the conventional antipsychotics. Anticholinergic effects can be particularly severe if used in the elderly or if low-potency agents are used in combination with other medications possessing this property, such as tricyclic antidepressants or antiparkinsonian agents.

Patients who are troubled by dry mouth should be advised to rinse their mouth out frequently with water and to chew sugar-free gum and candy to prevent fungal infections and dental caries. Oral lubricants (Xerolube) and ice chips are other treatments. If patients are experiencing constipation, the first treatment should be increases in fluid and dietary fiber intake and exercise, if possible. If not, constipation should be treated with routine laxative preparations, such as Metamucil or docusate sodium. Untreated constipation can lead to paralytic ileus, which may necessitate consultation or referral to outside specialists. Urinary retention may be treated with bethanechol (Urecholine), 20 to 40 mg/day. However, persistent anticholinergic effects probably warrant a decrease in antipsychotic dose or switching to another agent.

Marked anticholinergic effects may include:

- Cognitive decline
- Severe agitation
- Disorientation
- Hallucinations
- Seizures
- High fever
- Mydriasis.

If these signs or symptoms occur, the causative agent should be discontinued and the patient should be kept under close medical supervision.

■ Hematologic Effects

Leukopenia (white blood cell [WBC] count around $3500/mm^3$) is fairly common but not a clinically serious problem. If the WBC count is $<3000/mm^3$ or the absolute neutrophil count (ANC) is $<1000/mm^3$, the antipsychotic should be discontinued and the WBC should be monitored closely until it normalizes. Agranulocytosis is rare and reportedly occurs in 1/ 100,000 to 1/500,000 patients receiving traditional antipsychotics. It may occur most frequently with piperazine phenothiazines. The onset is usually within the first 3 months of therapy. If a patient develops signs and symptoms of infection, a WBC count with differential should be performed. Routine blood monitoring, however, is not indicated. Thrombocytopenia and pancytopenia have been reported to occur rarely.

■ Ophthalmic Side Effects

Secondary to anticholinergic effects of these medications, impairment in visual accommodation may result. This effect is usually temporary. Anticholinergic effects may also exacerbate narrow-angle glaucoma, which can result from increases in intraocular pressure. Higher-potency antipsychotics should be used in susceptible individuals.

Thioridazine is associated with irreversible pigmentation of the retina when given in doses >800 mg/day. The pigmentation is caused by melanin deposits and is similar to retinitis pigmentosa, possibly progressing to blindness even following thioridazine discontinuation. Therefore, patients taking this medication should be monitored for this effect and the drug should be discontinued if any changes in pigmentation occur. Opaque whitish-brown deposits in the cornea and lens may occur with phenothiazine treatment, visible only by slit-lamp examination. They may progress to yellowish-brown granules, often stellate in shape. Although visual acuity is not usually affected, periodic slit-lamp ophthalmologic examinations are recommended in patients receiving long-term treatment with phenothiazines.

■ Dermatologic Effects

Allergic reactions rarely occur and do so primarily within the first 8 weeks of treatment. Rashes of maculopapular, petechial, erythematous, and urticarial manifestations have all been reported. Conventional antipsychotic drugs are often found in high concentrations in the skin of people taking them. A photosensitivity reaction that resembles a severe sunburn can occur in patients taking phenothiazines. This group of antipsychotics directly absorbs ultraviolet light and energy, resulting in the formation of free radicals, which can cause damage to the skin. Exposure to sunlight should be limited to between 30 and 60 minutes, and patients should be educated about the use of maximal blocking sunscreens, protective clothing, hats, and sunglasses.

Blue-gray to purplish skin discoloration, usually in areas of the body exposed to sunlight, can occur in patients receiving chlorpromazine. The coloration may begin as a tan or golden brown color and then progress to gray, blue, or purple tones. This generally occurs in patients:

- Receiving higher doses
- On long-term therapy
- Concurrently with a corneal or lens pigmentation.

■ Hepatic Effects

Abnormalities in liver function tests (LFTs), such as elevated aminotransferase and alkaline phosphatase, may occur in up to 50% of patients on conventional antipsychotics. Generally, these elevations occur without clinical significance, although they should be routinely monitored. If LFTs are elevated to >3 times the upper limit of normal, the medication should be changed to a chemically unrelated agent.

Cholestatic hepatocellular jaundice occurs in approximately 2% of patients receiving phenothiazines, usually within the first 5 weeks of treatment. Prodromal symptoms often include:

- Malaise
- Fatigue
- Fever
- Chills
- Arthralgia
- Myalgia
- Gastrointestinal symptoms
- Severe pruritus.

The antipsychotic should be discontinued if jaundice occurs; once discontinued, symptoms usually disappear within 2 to 8 weeks. Pruritus may be palliatively treated with oral or topical antihistamines.

■ Epileptogenic Effects

Low-potency antipsychotic use may be associated with a slowing and an increased synchronization of the electroencephalogram (EEG). As a potential result, the lower-potency agents decrease the seizure threshold. Although this adverse effect is rare, administering a low-potency agent warrants consideration in patients with a seizure disorder or organic brain lesion.

■ Weight Gain

A common adverse effect of treatment with antipsychotics is weight gain, which can be significant in some cases. Weight gain may be mediated through blockade of the 5-hydroxytryptamine $(5\text{-HT})_{2C}$ receptors as well as H_1. Average weight gain is between 1.5 and 6.9 kg (3.3 and 15.2 lb) over 6 months of treatment with conventional agents. Molindone and perhaps loxapine do not cause as great a weight gain as do the other antipsychotics. Patients should be educated about the morbidity associated with increases in weight such as:

- Hypercholesterolemia
- Diabetes
- Orthopedic complications
- Coronary artery disease.

Treatment plans should include diet modification and exercise, if possible. Weight gain is one of the primary reasons for nonadherence in patients taking conventional antipsychotics.

■ Endocrine Effects/Sexual Dysfunction

Antagonism of dopamine receptors in the tuberofundibular tract results in increased secretion of prolactin. The main physiologic effects of increased prolactin are suppression of gonadal activity and induction of the synthesis and secretion of milk. All conventional antipsychotics trigger a sustained increase in prolactin release. In men, the most commonly reported sexual dysfunctions are disturbances of erection and ejaculation, occurring in 30% to 60% of males treated with conventional antipsychotics. Women most likely experience decreased libido and orgasmic dysfunction, including difficulty achieving orgasm, changes in the quality of orgasm, and anorgasmia. This prevalence is slightly lower than in men, between 25% and 30%. Clinicians may not learn about these adverse effects if they do not ask about them specifically. Women may also experience menstrual irregularities, including amenorrhea and changes in the quantity of menses. Between 50% and 90% of women taking conventional antipsychotics experience some menstrual irregularity. Antagonism of α_1 receptors and anticholinergic effects may also contribute to sexual dysfunction.

Treatment options include lowering the dosage or switching to an SGAD. Other drugs with anticholinergic properties should be discontinued. Bromocriptine, a dopamine agonist, has been used to improve libido in some patients in hyperprolactinemic states. Since other agents are available, eg, the SGADs, bromocriptine should generally not be used due to its ability to exacerbate psychoses and cause nausea and hypotension. Other endocrine side effects that may occur rarely include the inappropriate secretion of antidiuretic hormone and diabetes or impaired glucose tolerance.

■ **Neuroleptic Malignant Syndrome**
Neuroleptic malignant syndrome (NMS) is a life-threatening adverse effect of antipsychotic treatment. Mortality in well-developed cases ranges from 20% to 30%, although it may be much less according to recent studies. The clinical presentation of NMS evolves over 24 to 72 hours and usually includes:

- Severe muscular rigidity
- Autonomic instability:
  – Hyperthermia
  – Tachycardia
  – Increased blood pressure
  – Tachypnea
  – Diaphoresis
- Altered consciousness.

A patient with NMS usually presents with muscle rigidity that progresses to include an elevated temperature, fluctuating consciousness, and unstable vital signs. These symptoms are often associated with elevations in creatine phosphokinase. Liver transaminase elevations, myoglobinemia, myoglobinuria, and leukocytosis may occur, as well as renal failure. Early symptoms of agitation may be mistaken for increased psychosis. Levenson's diagnostic criteria, the most accepted in the field, are listed in Table 5.5. For purposes of diagnosis, the patient should have two major manifestations and four minor manifestations, with a clinical history suggestive of the possibility of NMS.

TABLE 5.5 — LEVENSON'S DIAGNOSTIC CRITERIA FOR NEUROLEPTIC MALIGNANT SYNDROME
Major Manifestations • Fever • Rigidity • Elevated creatine phosphokinase
Minor Manifestations • Tachycardia • Abnormal blood pressure • Tachypnea • Altered consciousness • Diaphoresis • Leukocytosis

Rapid dose escalation and the use of high-potency antipsychotics at higher doses are associated with a greater incidence of NMS. Younger age, dehydration, previous episodes of NMS, and male gender are also risk factors for the development of NMS. The diagnosis is often difficult to discern and may result as an exclusion from many other possibilities. Patients present quite differently and may not experience all of the hallmark signs and symptoms. Other possible causative conditions should be ruled out by differential diagnosis (Table 5.6).

5

TABLE 5.6 — DIFFERENTIAL DIAGNOSIS FOR NEUROLEPTIC MALIGNANT SYNDROME

- Malignant hyperthermia
- Lethal catatonia
- Heat stroke
- Severe extrapyramidal symptoms
- Parkinson's disease
- Central nervous system infection
- Allergic drug reactions
- Anticholinergic delirium
- Systemic infection
- Lithium toxicity

When NMS is diagnosed or suspected, antipsychotics should be discontinued and supportive and symptomatic treatment begun. This may include antipyretics, cooling blanket, intravenous fluids, oxygen, and adequate nutritional support. If a patient has a temperature greater than $101°$ F, treatment with dopamine agonists, such as bromocriptine, should be considered. The dose of bromocriptine is 2.5 mg po every 8 hours, increasing to a maximum of 60 mg/day. This should be continued for 10 days after the resolution of symptoms, then tapered off gradually. If such treatment is inadequate, dantrolene can be administered at 60 mg po every 6 hours. Liver transaminases should be monitored during therapy. After symptoms have resolved, patients should be treated with a different antipsychotic agent, avoiding high-potency and depot agents, if possible.

Use During Pregnancy and Lactation

The risk of teratogenesis with traditional antipsychotics is not well studied; however, its occurrence appears to be relatively low with the high-potency drugs. Haloperidol was once studied in the treatment of hyperemesis gravidarum without negative effects. Low-potency agents may be associated with a small increase in the relative risk for congenital anomalies. Altshuler and associates (1996) performed a meta-analysis of the effects of first-trimester exposure to low-potency antipsychotics and reported a baseline incidence of 2% increasing to 2.4% with treatment. Case reports have described limb malformations, but they appear to be rare. The risks of antipsychotic use must be weighed against the benefits of treatment. Clinicians may consider discontinuing antipsychotic drugs during the first trimester, but psychotic relapse in the mother can also be dangerous to the fetus. Antipsychotics are found in breast milk with the milk-to-plasma ratio of 0.5 to 1. Mothers who are being treated with traditional antipsychotics should not breast feed.

SUGGESTED READING

Altshuler LL, Cohen L, Szuba MP, Burt VK, Gitlin M, Mintz J. Pharmacologic management of psychiatric illness during pregnancy: dilemmas and guidelines. *Am J Psychiatry*. 1996;153:592-606.

McEvoy JP, Hogarty GE, Steingard S. Optimal dose of neuroleptic in acute schizophrenia. A controlled study of the neuroleptic threshold and higher haloperidol dose. *Arch Gen Psychiatry*. 1991; 48:739-745.

Schooler NR, Keith SJ, Severe JB, et al. Relapse and rehospitalization during maintenance treatment of schizophrenia. The effects of dose reduction and family treatment. *Arch Gen Psychiatry*. 1997;54:453-463.

Tandon R, Milner K, Jibson MD. Antipsychotics from theory to practice: integrating clinical and basic data. *J Clin Psychiatry*. 1999;60(suppl 8):21-28.

5

6

Extrapyramidal Symptoms/ Tardive Dyskinesia

Extrapyramidal symptoms (EPS), including akathisia, dystonia, and pseudoparkinsonism, are the major adverse effects associated with traditional antipsychotic therapy. These side effects are a result of dopamine antagonism in the nigrostriatal pathway. The rates of EPS with second-generation antipsychotic drugs (SGADs) are listed in Chapter 4, *Comparative Data Among Second-Generation Antipsychotic Drugs.*

Akathisia

Akathisia is the most frequently occurring of these adverse effects. Approximately 50% of patients treated with traditional agents will experience a subjective feeling of restlessness. These patients may pace, rock from foot to foot while standing, tap their feet, or move their feet restlessly while sitting. Frequently, patients complain that they are unable to feel comfortable regardless of what they do. Patients may feel anxious and irritable. Severe akathisia has resulted in aggressive and suicidal acts. The onset of akathisia is usually 5 to 10 days after the first dose or increase in dosage. Younger patients and those taking high doses of high-potency antipsychotics are at greater risk for the development of akathisia. This adverse effect may be difficult to diagnose and may be confused with anxiety, agitation, tardive dyskinesia, or a worsening of psychosis. The management of akathisia includes

- Reducing the antipsychotic dose
- Changing to another agent
- Use of lipid-soluble β-blocking agents or benzodiazepines.

Propranolol, between 30 and 120 mg/day, is highly effective for treatment, and relief is usually observed within 48 hours. Lorazepam (1 to 3 mg/day) and clonazepam (1 to 3 mg/day) may also be used for the treatment of akathisia. In general, SGADs cause less of this troubling side effect, but risperidone and olanzapine may be associated with this problem.

Dystonia

Acute dystonic reactions are abrupt in onset and are usually seen within 24 to 96 hours after a first dose or increase in dosage. Characteristic signs and symptoms may occur in 10% to 20% of patients and include abnormal positioning or spasm of the muscles of the head, neck, limbs, or trunk. Table 6.1 lists various forms of dystonia that may occur.

Risk factors for dystonia include:
- Young age
- African American race
- Patients with a history of acute dystonic reactions.

Dystonia almost always responds rapidly to antiparkinsonian medications and can usually be prevented either by pretreatment with these drugs or by limiting the neuroleptic dosage prescribed. Benztropine, 2 mg intramuscularly (IM), or diphenhydramine, 50 mg IM, will usually control the dystonia within 15 to 20 minutes. Response to oral administration of these agents will not occur for 30 to 40 minutes. If the initial dose does not provide control, another dose can be given in 30 minutes. Oral prophylaxis may include any of the anticholinergic medications listed in Table 6.2. If prophylaxis is used in a high-risk patient, its use should be reevaluated once the patient is stabilized on the antipsychotic. The incidence of dystonia is much less

TABLE 6.1 — FORMS OF DYSTONIA	
Form of Dystonia	**Signs and Symptoms**
Blepharospasm	Involuntary tight contraction of the eyelids
Dysarthria	Unclear pronunciation or speech
Dysphagia	Difficulty in swallowing
Grimacing	Spasms of facial and jaw muscles
Macroglossia	Thickened or slurred speech due to hypertonic or enlarged tongue
Oculogyric crisis	Eyes deviated upward, downward, or sideways
Opisthotonos	Arching backward of the head, neck, and spine
Pharyngeal/laryngeal dystonia	Spasm of the throat, difficulty breathing
Tongue protrusion/ glossospasm	Spastic movements of the tongue
Torticollis/retrocollis	Abnormal positioning of the head and neck in relation to the rest of body
Trismus	Spasm of the jaw muscles, keeping the jaws tightly closed

with the SGADs, but dystonic reactions have been reported with risperidone and olanzapine.

Pseudoparkinsonism

Pseudoparkinsonism resembles idiopathic Parkinson's disease and occurs in approximately 15% of patients treated with traditional antipsychotics. The onset of symptoms is usually seen within 1 to 2 weeks following initiation or a dose increase. Risk factors include:

TABLE 6.2 — DOSING RANGES FOR ANTICHOLINERGICS

Generic (Trade) Name	Usual Dose Range
Amantadine (Symmetrel)	100 mg bid-tid
Benztropine (Cogentin)	1-2 mg bid
Biperiden (Akineton)	1-3 mg bid
Diphenhydramine (Benadryl)	25-50 mg bid
Orphenadrine (Norflex)	100 mg bid
Procyclidine (Kemadrin)	2.5-5 mg tid
Trihexyphenidyl (Artane)	1-3 mg tid

- Older age
- Female gender
- High doses
- Possibly those with depressive symptoms.

A patient may have any of the four cardinal symptoms listed in Table 6.3.

The management of pseudoparkinsonism includes a dose reduction, switching to a different agent, or the use of anticholinergic or dopaminergic drugs. Any of the anticholinergic agents listed in Table 6.2 are effective for relieving parkinsonlike symptoms. Benztropine has a longer half-life, thus allowing twice-daily dosing. Trihexyphenidyl has more abuse potential, whereas diphenhydramine produces more sedation than the other agents. With all of these treatments, symptoms will usually resolve in 3 to 4 days, but a minimum of at least 2 weeks of treatment is normally required for complete response. Amantadine is as effective as other anticholinergic agents, with significantly less effect on memory function. Dosage adjustment is necessary with renal insufficiency, and livedo reticularis may occur in 1% to 5% of patients.

TABLE 6.3 — CARDINAL SYMPTOMS OF PSEUDOPARKINSONISM

- Akinesia, bradykinesia, or decreased motor activity including difficulty initiating movement and extreme slowness, masklike facial expression, micrographia, slowed speech, and decreased arm swing
- Tremor, known as pill-rolling type, predominant at rest, decreases with movement, usually involves the fingers and hands, although it may be seen in the arms, legs, neck, head, and chin (it may often be activated by having the patient perform mechanical movements with one extremity, 4 to 7 cycles/sec)
- Cogwheel rigidity, seen as the patient's limbs yield in jerky, ratchetlike fashion when passively moved by the examiner (a mild form may present as stiffness)
- Postural abnormalities and instability manifested as stooped posture, difficulty in maintaining stability when changing body position, and a gait that ranges from slow and shuffling to festinating (a result of dysfunction in autonomic stability combined with a shift in the center of gravity due to the stooped posture)

Some patients may experience a reduction in benefit after 1 to 3 months of amantadine treatment.

Tardive Dyskinesia

■ Epidemiology

Tardive dyskinesia (TD) is a syndrome characterized by abnormal choreiform (rapid, objectively, purposeless, irregular, and spontaneous) and athetoid (slow and irregular) movements occurring late in onset in relation to initiation of antipsychotic therapy. This adverse effect usually develops over several months and occurs after at least 3 months of conventional antipsychotic treatment. The estimated average prevalence is 20%, with a range of 13% to 36%. The incidence of new cases per treatment year is approximately 5%. The incidence with SGADs is <2%. TD is reversible in one third to one half of cases with the discontinuance of the antipsychotic. When the antipsychotic is tapered or discontinued, there is usually worsening of abnormal movements initially. Risk factors include:

- Older age
- Duration of antipsychotic treatment
- Higher rates of EPS
- Substance abuse
- Mood disorders.

■ Signs and Symptoms

The characteristic signs and symptoms usually involve a buccolingual-masticatory syndrome or orofacial movements. Typically, these are the first detectable signs of TD and can progress to movements severe enough to interfere with chewing, speech, respiration, or swallowing. These include:

- Lip smacking
- Puckering
- Sucking
- Pouting
- Tongue writhing, protrusion, and tremor.

Other facial movements include frequent blinking, grimacing, and tics. Truncal and limb movements usually are seen as TD progresses. This includes twisting, spreading, flexion and extension of the fingers, and toe dorsiflexion. Unusual posture, hyperextension, pelvic thrusting, exaggerated lordosis (bending backward), rocking, and swaying may all occur in the truncal area. While younger adults report more truncal movements, older patients experience more orofacial movements. Voluntary attempts to suppress the movements usually work temporarily but may actually lead to worsening of the symptoms.

■ Pathophysiology

The pathophysiology of TD is complex and has not been satisfactorily explained. The original theory involves dopamine supersensitivity of striatal dopamine receptors due to long-term antipsychotic treatment. This, however, does not entirely explain the pathogenesis of TD. This may partially be true, but depletion of gamma-aminobutyric acid (GABA) may also play a role. Decreased GABA turnover or binding sites may occur after chronic antipsychotic exposure, leading to increased inhibition of GABAergic outflow. This results in a loss of inhibition to the thalamocortical projections. Increased activity may lead to blockade of dopamine $(D)_2$ projections. Other neurotransmitters and neuropeptides such as cholecystokinin may play a role in the etiology, and changes at the N-methyl-D-aspartate (NMDA) and opiate receptors may be involved.

■ Treatment

Dosage reduction may decrease or eliminate symptoms in some patients. However, the development of TD is a medical, legal, and ethical problem. If patients with TD are kept on antipsychotic therapy, there is the possibility of symptoms worsening. Prevention of this adverse effect is important. Patients with clear target symptoms should be treated at the minimum effective dose. Regular examinations and assessments should be done to ensure that patients do not have signs and symptoms. Switching to or initiating therapy with an SGAD may prevent TD, since these drugs appear to involve a lower incidence of this problem. Minimizing the use of anticholinergics is also important. There are no Food and Drug Administration–approved agents for the treatment of TD. Many therapies have been tried with little success. Benzodiazepines, such as clonazepam, are sometimes initially effective but usually lose efficacy by 3 to 4 months. Valproate and baclofen have also been used with modest results. Dopamine-depleting agents, such as reserpine and methyldopa, may alleviate symptoms in some patients but have many serious side effects associated with their use. Calcium channel blockers and botulinus toxin have also been tried with few positive effects. Vitamin E has been tried in several double-blind trials with mixed results. The dose range usually used is 1200 to 1600 IU for 4 to 12 weeks. Vitamin E may be more effective in patients who have had TD for <5 years. Nonetheless, the beneficial effects of vitamin E are modest.

Clozapine may be effective in ameliorating existing TD. Patients with moderate to severe TD will usually have marked improvements in their symptoms when changed to clozapine from conventional antipsychotics. However, approximately 9 to 10 months of clozapine treatment may be required before the symptoms of TD begin to remit. The American Psychiatric Association Task Force on Tardive Dyskinesia (1992) issued recommendations for the prevention and management of TD (Table 6.4).

TABLE 6.4 — PREVENTION AND MANAGEMENT OF TARDIVE DYSKINESIA

- Establish objective evidence that antipsychotic medications are effective for an individual
- Use the lowest effective dose of antipsychotic
- Prescribe cautiously to children, elderly people, and individuals with mood disorders
- Examine patients on a regular basis for evidence of tardive dyskinesia
- When tardive dyskinesia is diagnosed, consider alternatives to antipsychotics, obtain informed consent, and also consider dosage reduction
- If the tardive dyskinesia worsens, consider a number of options, including discontinuing the antipsychotics, switching to a different drug, or initiating a trial of clozapine

---

SUGGESTED READING

Akiyama K. Algorithms for neuroleptic-associated tardive movement disorders. *Psychiatry Clin Neurosci*. 1999;53(suppl): S23-S29.

Casey DE. Effects of clozapine therapy in schizophrenic individuals at risk for tardive dyskinesia. *J Clin Psychiatry*. 1998;59(suppl 3):31-37.

Casey DE. Tardive dyskinesia and atypical antipsychotic drugs. *Schizophr Res*. 1999;35(suppl):S61-S66.

Collaborative Working Group on Clinical Trial Evaluations. Assessment of EPS and tardive dyskinesia in clinical trials. *J Clin Psychiatry*. 1998;59(suppl 12):23-27.

Gerlach J. The continuing problem of extrapyramidal symptoms: strategies for avoidance and effective treatment. *J Clin Psychiatry*. 1999;60(suppl 23):20-24.

Gupta S, Mosnik D, Black DW, Berry S, Masand PS. Tardive dyskinesia: review of treatments past, present, and future. *Ann Clin Psychiatry*. 1999;11:257-266.

Lader M. Some adverse effects of antipsychotics: prevention and treatment. *J Clin Psychiatry*. 1999;60(suppl 12):18-21.

Van Putten T, Marder SR. Behavioral toxicity of antipsychotic drugs. *J Clin Psychiatry*. 1987;48(suppl):13-19.

7 Metabolic Effects of Antipsychotic Drugs

People with schizophrenia have a shortened life span as compared with the general population, with excess mortality due to both natural and unnatural causes. This may partially be explained by the fact that many people have concomitant illnesses, such as type 2 diabetes mellitus (DM) and cardiovascular disorders, that constitute the metabolic syndrome in which the phenotype is excess visceral fat distribution. The mechanism of this syndrome is unclear, but we know that antipsychotic treatment may compound or exacerbate metabolic issues such as weight gain, glucose regulation, and lipid abnormalities.

Weight Gain

Currently in the United States, one half of adults are overweight (body-mass index [BMI] ≥ 25 kg/m^2) and one fifth of the population is considered obese (BMI ≥ 30 kg/m^2). BMI among people with schizophrenia, however, exceeds the general population estimates. Many psychiatric patients, including those with schizophrenia, have excess adipose tissue that is often centrally distributed. Central adipose tissue exhibits higher metabolic activity than peripheral tissue. In general, obesity increases the risk for a myriad of medical disorders (Table 7.1). People with schizophrenia exhibit high relative rates of smoking and drug abuse, and have several medical disorders that also compound the high rates of morbidity and mortality seen in this population.

TABLE 7.1 — CLINICAL CONSEQUENCES OF WEIGHT GAIN

- Hypertension
- Atherosclerosis
- Type 2 diabetes
- Cardiovascular disease
- Stroke
- Cancer:
  - Endometrial
  - Breast
  - Prostate
  - Colon
- Osteoarthritis
- Sleep apnea
- Nonadherence to medication
- Impairment of quality of life
- Social withdrawal

■ Mechanism of Weight Gain

Body weight is dependent on a balance between the intake and expenditure of energy. Although behavioral, environmental, and neurochemical factors play critical roles in energy intake and expenditure, heritability studies suggest that up to 70% of body weight is genetically mediated. Antipsychotic medications are associated with differing degrees of weight gain, and although the mechanism is not completely clear, most reports have emphasized that changes occur in putative neurocircuits that participate in increased energy intake (eg, increased appetite). Many patients experiencing weight gain during antipsychotic treatment report decreased satiety and increased:

- Appetite
- Binge eating
- Carbohydrate craving
- Food preference changes.

Serotonin has a well-known effect on satiety. Relative increases in serotonin have been shown to decrease feeding behavior, while antagonism of serotonin stimulates increased energy intake. Serotonin$_{2C}$ receptors have been under investigation as candidate receptors for psychotropic-induced weight gain. While much evidence suggest that antagonists at this receptor have weight-gain liabilities, other reports have failed to correlate weight gain with 5HT$_{2C}$ affinity. Additionally, ziprasidone, which is associated with minimal weight gain, exhibits high *in vivo* activity for the 5HT$_{2C}$ receptor.

Dopamine or noradrenaline antagonism at the lateral hypothalamus may affect satiety. Many other neurotransmitters, neuropeptides, and cytokines may play a role in mediating weight gain. Prolactin, leptin, GABA agonists, neuropeptide Y, and tumor necrosis factor alpha are a few that may be involved to some degree. Histamine also signals the hypothalamus, and histamine antagonism stimulates energy intake centrally by increasing appetite. A robust correlation between the affinity of second-generation antipsychotic drugs (SGAD) for histamine receptors and antipsychotic-induced weight gain has been reported.

■ Comparative Weight Gain

Many studies describe weight gain among people taking various antipsychotic agents. The most comprehensive report to date is a meta-analysis of over 80 studies (Figure 7.1). Weight gain is highly variable among antipsychotics. Two SGADs, olanzapine and clozapine, appear to be associated with the highest degree of weight gain (4 to 4.5 kg over 10 weeks). Low-potency antipsychotics, such as chlorpromazine and thioridazine, are associated with high weight gains, possibly relating to their high degree of histamine blockade. In recent years, a metric from the American Heart Association describing weight gain that has become popular is calculating the percentage of people who gain >7% of their baseline weight (Table 7.2).

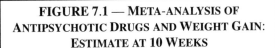

FIGURE 7.1 — META-ANALYSIS OF ANTIPSYCHOTIC DRUGS AND WEIGHT GAIN: ESTIMATE AT 10 WEEKS

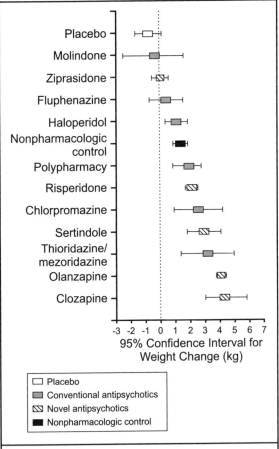

Adapted from: Allison DB, et al. *Am J Psychiatry.* 1999; 156:1686-1696.

TABLE 7.2 — PERCENTAGE OF PATIENTS WITH ≥7% INCREASE IN BODY WEIGHT FROM PIVOTAL TRIALS		
Antipsychotic Drug	**Increase (%)**	
	Drug	**Placebo**
Aripiprazole	8	3
Ziprasidone	10	4
Risperidone	18	9
Quetiapine	25	4
Olanzapine	29	3

The time course for weight gain among individuals is less well described. Olanzapine weight gains at doses of 12.5 to 17.5 mg/day have been found to average 12 kg after 1 year of use. Weight gain with risperidone appears to plateau early in treatment and remains at about 2 to 3 kg at 1 year. Long-term data for quetiapine appear to demonstrate similar weight gain to that with risperidone. Ziprasidone is associated with no or minimal weight gain in patients followed for up to 1 year. Aripiprazole is associated with about 1 kg weight gain in patients treated 6 to 12 months. Most data imply that weight gain is generally not dose dependent with the SGADs and that patients with low BMIs may gain the most weight.

■ **Management of Weight Gain**

Patients should be counseled and well-informed about the risk of body weight increase with antipsychotic treatment. High-calorie food and beverage intake should be minimized, as well as the consumption of fat reduced. Weight should be regularly monitored and realistic weight targets should be a part of long-term management. Physical activity should be recommended and patients should be advised to exercise regularly. Weight-control groups or individual behavioral therapy sessions may be helpful for obesity-prone patients. Table 7.3 lists clinical implications of weight gain.

TABLE 7.3 — CLINICAL IMPLICATIONS OF ANTIPSYCHOTIC-INDUCED WEIGHT GAIN IN PATIENTS WITH SCHIZOPHRENIA

Screening Measures
- Baseline weight
- Weight and weight-related laboratory parameters (glucose, triglycerides, total high- and low-density lipoprotein cholesterol)
- Risk factors for diabetes mellitus and cardiovascular disease
- Additional risk factors:
  – Smoking
  – Substance abuse (alcohol and/or drugs)
- Hemoglobin A_{1C} level

Management Strategies
- Nonpharmacologic options:
  – Diet
  – Exercise
  – Behavioral therapy
- Pharmacologic options:
  – Dose reduction
  – Change of antipsychotic medication
  – Weight-reduction drugs, in selected cases

Kurzthaler I, Fleischhacker WW. The clinical implications of weight gain in schizophrenia. *J Clin Psychiatry*. 2001;62(suppl 7):32-37.

Lowering the dose of antipsychotics may be helpful for curbing weight gain in some patients; however, many data suggest that weight gain is not dose related. The risk of symptom exacerbation or relapse is an issue if dosing is lowered. Those at high risk for weight gain or weight-related problems should initially be given drugs with a low weight-gain liability. Switching patients from an antipsychotic that has caused weight gain to another agent may be beneficial for weight control.

The use of weight-reducing drugs for antipsychotic-induced weight gain is controversial and understudied. There have been several reports of psychosis associated with the use of fenfluramine and/or phenteramine. Orlistat and sibutramine are Food and Drug Administration (FDA)–approved weight-loss agents in the United States, but neither has been systematically studied for antipsychotic-induced weight gain. Orlistat is an *ex vivo* agent with minimal systemic absorption that blocks pancreatic and gastric lipases. Sibutramine is a mixed serotonergic and noradrenergic reuptake inhibitor. Small studies of sibutramine have not been promising as weight loss rates have been similar to placebo values. Nizatadine, amantadine, and topiramate have also been used, but data as to the safety and efficacy of these medications are lacking. Moreover, trials using topiramate for weight loss in schizophrenia have recently been halted because patients developed:

- Memory problems
- Excessive fatigue
- Numbness and tingling in the limbs
- Insomnia.

Therefore, weight-reduction drugs do not appear to be of great benefit and may have a high risk-to-benefit profile. Nonpharmacologic options appear to offer better outcomes for weight loss.

Glucose Dysregulation

Metabolic disturbances in psychotic patients, particularly impaired glucose metabolism, were first described in psychotic patients prior to the introduction of antipsychotic medications. Also, the risk for type 2

DM may be higher in schizophrenic patients compared with the general population, which predisposes some schizophrenic patients to have glucose dysregulation during antipsychotic treatment. Antipsychotic medications themselves have been associated with:

- Impaired glucose metabolism
- Exacerbation of existing type 1 and 2 diabetes
- New-onset type 2 DM
- Diabetic ketoacidosis (DKA).

Clozapine, olanzapine, and chlorpromazine have been implicated as having the highest associated likelihood of DM occurrence. Abdominal or central adiposity may contribute to glucose dysregulation. However, DM may occur with olanzapine and clozapine independent of weight change.

■ Diagnostic Classification

The American Diabetes Association has developed new diagnostic criteria for DM (Table 7.4). Additionally, impaired glucose tolerance (IGT) (fasting plasma glucose >110 mg/dL and <126 mg/dL or 2-hour postload glucose >140 mg/dL and <200 mg/dL) is present in approximately 20 million people. This prediabetic condition has a 5% to 10% annual risk of converting to DM. One hypothesis as to why patients develop DM soon after antipsychotic initiation is that they may have had undiagnosed IGT or DM prior to treatment. Thus careful baseline measurements and histories should be taken prior to starting medication.

■ Mechanism of Action

Prior to the introduction of antipsychotics, some patients with schizophrenia showed a delay in the return of blood sugar to a normal level after administration of an intravenous dextrose solution. Early on, this was hypothesized to be caused by a low insulin level in the blood, slow metabolism of insulin, or the

TABLE 7.4 — AMERICAN DIABETES ASSOCIATION DIAGNOSTIC CRITERIA FOR DIABETES MELLITUS

Biochemical Index	Normal Value	Diagnostic Criteria
Hemoglobin A_{1C} (%)	<6	NA
Fasting plasma glucose (mg/dL)	<110	≥126
Plasma glucose 2 hours after a 75g oral glucose tolerance test (mg/dL)	<140	≥200

Abbreviation: NA, not an acceptable instrument for diagnosing diabetes.

American Diabetes Association. *Diabetes Care*. 2001;24: S33-S49.

overactivity of some product of the endocrine system that inhibits the production of normal insulin. A characteristic feature of patients with IGT, particularly those with type 2 DM, is insulin resistance. Insulin resistance and decreased insulin secretion are due to decreased pancreatic β-cell function in the development of type 2 DM. Some evidence suggests that clozapine and olanzapine are also associated with insulin resistance independent of differences in adiposity. Resistance to insulin can develop due to numerous abnormalities in the signaling pathway. SGADs may:

- Cause insulin resistance directly by altering binding characteristics
- Reduce the number or half-life of glucose transporters
- Interfere with the transportation of glucose from the microsome to the plasma membrane.

Increased insulin secretion due to weight gain may be a mediating factor for hyperglycemia in people treated with SGADs. The relative risk of developing type 2

DM increases with significant gain in weight similar to that seen with some antipsychotic agents (Figure 7.2). Cases of type 2 DM have rarely been reported with drugs that have a low weight-gain liability.

■ Comparative Risk of Diabetes

Through 2001, at least 45 case reports have been reported in the literature detailing new-onset type 2 DM and DKA occurring in patients treated with SGADs. Twenty (44%) and 19 (42%) of the cases were for clozapine and olanzapine, respectively. Only three cases each have been reported for risperidone and quetiapine, and no cases to date have been published for ziprasidone or aripiprazole. From these reports, it appears that men and blacks may be at higher risk for the development of DM. Also, while the majority of cases occurred in people who were overweight prior to treatment, 50% of those who developed DM did not experience weight gain during therapy. During short-term trials with most SGADs, fasting blood glucose (FBG) has not been noted to significantly rise. Fasting plasma insulin levels, however, appear to significantly increase with olanzapine and clozapine, demonstrating these drugs' immediate effects on glucose regulation. In longer-term studies, FBG is noted to significantly rise with clozapine and olanzapine. During long-term studies, it appears that approximately one third of patients treated with clozapine for up to 5 years will develop DM. Long-term studies on the incidence of DM for the other SGADs are lacking as are trials determining the relative risk for developing DM for each SGAD.

■ Diabetic Ketoacidosis

Diabetic ketoacidosis has been a presenting symptom in at least 10 reported cases during clozapine treatment and at least five case reports with olanzapine therapy. DKA occurs when insulin is not present for the body to use glucose. Metabolism of fat occurs, pro-

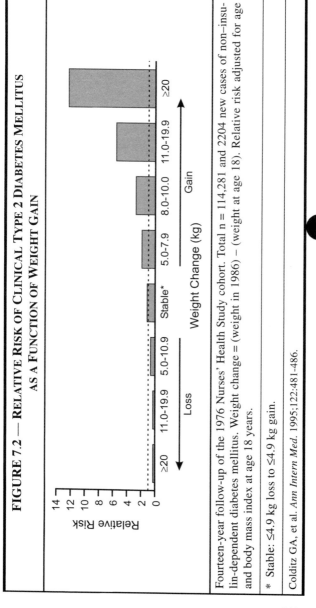

FIGURE 7.2 — **RELATIVE RISK OF CLINICAL TYPE 2 DIABETES MELLITUS AS A FUNCTION OF WEIGHT GAIN**

Fourteen-year follow-up of the 1976 Nurses' Health Study cohort. Total n = 114,281 and 2204 new cases of non–insulin-dependent diabetes mellitus. Weight change = (weight in 1986) – (weight at age 18). Relative risk adjusted for age and body mass index at age 18 years.

* Stable: ≤4.9 kg loss to ≤4.9 kg gain.

Colditz GA, et al. *Ann Intern Med.* 1995;122:481-486.

ducing excess ketones, which contribute to blood becoming more acidic than body tissues. Patients usually present with:

- Polyuria
- Nausea
- Vomiting
- Abdominal pain.

Lethargy or somnolence is common later in development of DKA and in untreated patients, and it may progress to coma. In patients with no history of type 1 DM, DKA may not be considered initially. Since the patient may not volunteer a history of polyuria, DKA may be mistaken for many other ailments. Signs of dehydration are usually present, and some patients are hypotensive. Kussmaul's respiration (a distinctive pattern of slow, deep breaths) may be present, and acetone may be detected on the breath. Blood glucose levels are typically >300 mg/dL as well as electrolyte imbalance and low plasma pH. Mortality from DKA is about 2%, and deaths have occurred from DKA as a presenting symptom of DM during both clozapine and olanzapine treatment.

■ Management

If hyperglycemia develops during treatment with SGADs, the patient's FBG level should be measured. If the results are questionable, a glucose tolerance test should be performed. Alternatives for therapy include continuing with the same antipsychotic medication together with an antiglycemic drug regimen or switching to a different antipsychotic. There are reports of people recovering from new-onset DM after withdrawal of olanzapine and clozapine. Switching patients to quetiapine, aripiprazole, ziprasidone, or risperidone may have positive effects on weight and glucose homeostasis, but few data are available for sequential use or effects of switching antipsychotic medications. In addition, there are no guidelines or recommendations for glycemic control in patients with schizophrenia who develop DM. Choices include insulin secretagogues (sulfonylurea or meglitinide) and insulin sensitizers (metformin or glitazone). Combination therapy is usually initiated if monotherapy fails to decrease FBG to <160 mg/dL. Patients should be regularly monitored for FBG and glycosylated hemoglobin (HbA_{1C}) during treatment.

Hyperlipidemia

Increases in plasma lipid levels have been noted with the phenothiazines, but negligible effects on lipids have occurred with the higher-potency agents such as haloperidol. Early on, clozapine was noted to cause a profound increase in serum triglycerides as well as a small increase in total cholesterol levels. Some evidence suggests that many patients with schizophrenia have high triglyceride levels prior to initiation of SGADs, which may indicate a possible underlying disorder of lipid metabolism exacerbated by antipsychotic agents. A typical increase in triglycerides during long-term treatment with olanzapine is about 60 to 70 mg/dL. A recent 6-week, comparative study of ziprasidone vs olanzapine found a 26 mg/dL increase in triglyceride levels with olanzapine, while a decrease was seen with ziprasidone. A few reports of elevated triglyceride levels have been reported with quetiapine. Ziprasidone treatment has been associated with lowering or normalization of triglycerides and total cholesterol following other antipsychotic medications. Risperidone and aripiprazole appear to have neutral effects on plasma lipid levels, including triglycerides and total cholesterol.

Clinical Monitoring

Baseline body weight, FBG, and lipid levels should be established and recorded before prescribing antipsychotic medications. All patients receiving clozapine or olanzapine should undergo monthly monitoring for 6 months. Longer indices of blood glucose concentration such as HBA_{1C} may be helpful in determining the effects of these medications on glucose tolerance. Monitoring for metabolic variables for other SGADs should be performed every 4 to 6 months.

SUGGESTED READING

Allison DB, Casey DE. Antipsychotic-induced weight gain: a review of the literature. *J Clin Psychiatry.* 2001;62(suppl 7):22-31.

Haupt DW, Newcomer JW. Hyperglycemia and antipsychotic medications. *J Clin Psychiatry.* 2001; 62(suppl 27):15-26.

Henderson DC, Cagliero E, Gray C, et al. Clozapine, diabetes mellitus, weight gain, and lipid abnormalities: a five-year naturalistic study. *Am J Psychiatry.* 2000;157:975-981.

Jin H, Meyer JM, Jeste DV. Phenomenology of and risk factors for new-onset diabetes mellitus and diabetic ketoacidosis associated with atypical antipsychotics: an analysis of 45 published cases. *Ann Clin Psychiatry.* 2002;14:59-64.

Liebzeit KA, Markowitz JS, Caley CF. New onset diabetes and atypical antipsychotics. *Eur Neuropsychopharmacol.* 2001; 11:25-32.

McIntyre RS, McCann SM, Kennedy SH. Antipsychotic metabolic effects: weight gain, diabetes mellitus, and lipid abnormalities. *Can J Psychiatry.* 2001;46:273-281.

Ryan MC, Thakore JH. Physical consequences of schizophrenia and its treatment. The metabolic syndrome. *Life Sci.* 2002;71:239-257.

8

Management of Acute Psychosis, Psychiatric Emergencies, and Aggressive/Suicidal Behavior

Psychiatric Emergencies and Acute Psychosis

Psychiatric emergencies are often found in the emergency department but may also occur in the psychiatric unit, in a medical facility, or in the outpatient setting. Most psychiatric emergencies require both pharmacologic and psychotherapeutic intervention. Often the psychiatrist must make decisions based on limited information or history. Each state has a statute that requires a physician to detain patients involuntarily in a psychiatric facility if the patient is judged to be dangerous to self or others. Patients who do not take care of their physical needs secondary to their psychosis, but are nonviolent, may still represent a threat to themselves or others, but this decision is often based on clinical judgment. Psychiatric patients who are considered dangerous may be legally detained and treated against their will; however, in most states, they cannot be chronically medicated without their consent unless a court order is obtained.

The two medications most often used for acute agitation are lorazepam and haloperidol. Either of these drugs can be given intravenously but are generally given by intramuscular (IM) injection (Table 8.1). Either medication is useful in ameliorating acute psychosis. Lorazepam is much better tolerated by patients than haloperidol. This is crucial, since patients will tend to resist the use of lorazepam much less than haloperidol, further enhancing its usefulness in acute care.

TABLE 8.1 — DOSES OF MEDICATIONS FOR PSYCHIATRIC EMERGENCIES AND ACUTE PSYCHOSIS

Drug	Dose
Lorazepam (Ativan)	1-2 mg IM q hour prn
Haloperidol (Haldol)	5-10 mg IM twice daily

Current recommendations advocate the use of IM lorazepam instead of IM haloperidol.

Intramuscular chlorpromazine and diazepam injections have also been used in the past, although diazepam is erratically absorbed from the deltoid muscle and chlorpromazine is associated with marked orthostatic hypotension and burning upon injection. Haloperidol may cause extrapyramidal symptoms (EPS), such as dystonic reactions, that can be particularly distressing, and an experience like this may cause the patient to avoid acute care. Haloperidol and chlorpromazine injections are more bioavailable than when the drugs are given orally; thus higher doses will reach systemic circulation better with injections than orally. Haloperidol is about 50% bioavailable; thus 10 mg orally is equivalent to a 5-mg IM injection. Chlorpromazine is about 25% bioavailable, with 100 mg orally being similar to a 25-mg IM injection. When EPS occur, anticholinergic agents should be given parenterally (see Chapter 6, *Extrapyramidal Symptoms/Tardive Dyskinesia*).

Treatment for acute schizophrenic exacerbation has changed in the past decade. Rapid tranquilization (neuroleptization) with antipsychotics, such as haloperidol in 5-mg doses administered every hour as needed, has been replaced by 10 to 20 mg/day of haloperidol or the acute use of second-generation antipsychotic drugs (SGADs) in combination with a benzodiazepine (usually lorazepam) as needed. Benzodiazepine augmentation of SGADs has been shown to control agitation as well as IM haloperidol during exacerbations of schizophrenia, and it is much better tolerated.

Intramuscular Second-Generation Antipsychotic Drugs

Recently IM ziprasidone was approved for rapid control of agitated behavior and psychotic symptoms in patients with acute exacerbations of schizophrenia. This is the only available IM formulation of an SGAD. At least five trials consisting of approximately 1000 patients have been completed to date. The recommended dosage is 10 to 20 mg administered as required, with a maximum dose of 40 mg/day. Doses of 10 mg may be administered every 2 hours; doses of 20 mg may be administered every 4 hours up to a maximum of 40 mg/day. Intramuscular ziprasidone is recommended to be used for <3 days and oral ziprasidone should be substituted as soon as possible. Ziprasidone was found to exhibit comparable to superior efficacy as compared with IM haloperidol. Continued benefits and clinical improvements in symptoms were noted after switching patients to oral ziprasidone.

Intramuscular ziprasidone is well tolerated and has demonstrated a favorable safety profile in short-term studies. The most common adverse events include:

- Nausea
- Headache
- Dizziness
- Anxiety
- Somnolence
- Insomnia
- Injection site pain.

Extrapyramidal side effects were generally low and significantly lower than those with IM haloperidol. In trials, approximately 8% of patients had QTc increases of 30 msec. Less than 2%, however, had QTc increases >450 msec. Hypertension was observed in about 7% of patients. Studies evaluating the switch between IM and oral ziprasidone noted higher rates of QTc prolongation during the switch. Nineteen percent of patients had 30-msec increases; however, <1% were 450 msec.

Concomitant benzodiazepine has been safely administered for additional sedation. Also, IM doses of ziprasidone up to 80 mg/day have been safely used. IM ziprasidone should be used with caution in the elderly and in patients with poor nutritional status and/or who are chronic drug and alcohol users. IM ziprasidone may not be a good selection in patients with existing cardiac disease or those taking metabolic inhibitors or other drugs that may prolong the QTc interval. Additionally, renal and hepatic impairment may preclude IM ziprasidone use until more safety data are available. Short-acting IM formulations of olanzapine and aripiprazole are currently under study as well.

Aggressive Behavior

Between 10% and 12% of patients with schizophrenia or major affective disorder may exhibit violent or aggressive behavior. Persistent, overt physical aggression is dangerous to both the victims and the perpetrators. In clinical practice, aggressive patients have often been treated with higher doses of antipsychotic medications, but this therapeutic approach has not been proven effective. In fact, higher doses may cause akathisia and irritability that may lead to increased aggressive behavior. Other pharmacologic strategies that have been used with varying results include anticonvulsants, benzodiazepines, serotonin reuptake inhibitors, and β-blocking agents. Additionally, some medications may cause aggressive behavior. Table 8.2

lists medications that have been linked to aggressive behavior.

TABLE 8.2 — MEDICATIONS LINKED TO AGGRESSIVE BEHAVIOR	
Drug Class	**Specific Agents**
Sedatives/anxiolytics	Alcohol, benzodiazepines, sedative anticonvulsants (eg, phenobarbital)
Stimulants	Cocaine, amphetamines, phenylpropanolamine
Antidepressants	Tricyclics, fluoxetine, fluvoxamine
Miscellaneous	Marijuana, anabolic steroids

The SGADs have been shown to decrease some aggressive behavior. Currently, clozapine appears to be the first choice in aggression treatment, with demonstrated efficacy in over 10 studies. These effects on aggressive behavior may be specific in that they are not mediated by sedation and are relatively independent of its general antipsychotic effect. Studies have found clozapine to decrease violent episodes, decrease the need for seclusion, and decrease hostility as measured by Brief Psychiatric Rating Scale (BPRS) hostility scores. Clozapine patients demonstrated the antiaggressive effects within 6 months of initiation, in some cases becoming less aggressive during the first few weeks. A treatment duration of 6 months, however, is recommended to induce a stable reduction of physical and verbal aggression. A few controlled clinical trials have examined risperidone vs conventional antipsychotics or placebo in regard to hostility as measured by these items on the BPRS or Positive and Negative Syndrome Scale. Risperidone has been shown to be superior to placebo and appears to offer benefits compared with those of conventional antipsychotics. Risperidone has been found to exert this effect independent of other symptoms. Several open reports have shown decreases in the need for seclusion and restraints as well. Quetiapine and olanzapine may offer benefits as well but have been reported only sparsely in the literature. It is unknown as to the antiaggressive effects of ziprasidone and aripiprazole. Of the antipsychotics currently available, clozapine may offer the most benefits for patients who are persistently aggressive.

Treatment of Suicidal Behavior

Suicide is the chief cause of premature death in individuals with schizophrenia. Between 20% and 40% of schizophrenic patients will attempt suicide at some point in their lifetime, and approximately 10% will die by this means. Risk factors identified in patients with schizophrenia are listed in Table 8.3.

In conjunction with other treatments, antipsychotic medications are commonly used to decrease the risk of suicide in patients with schizophrenia. Although there has been much inconsistency in the literature pertaining to conventional agents and suicide risk, treatment with recommended doses of these agents may be effective in decreasing suicide attempts. However, patients on extremely low or high doses have been found to have a higher likelihood of committing suicide. This is most likely due to EPS (particularly akathisia) and tardive dyskinesia (TD) at higher doses and to lack of efficacy at lower doses.

Several studies have examined clozapine and its effect on suicide attempts. Clozapine has been found to reduce the rate of suicide attempts as well as decrease the seriousness and lethality of attempts perhaps by as much as 75% to 85%. Mortality rates have been found to be lower during clozapine use than during

TABLE 8.3 — RISK FACTORS FOR SUICIDE IN PEOPLE WITH SCHIZOPHRENIA

Category	Risk Factor
Gender	Male
Race	White
Marital status	Never married, divorced, or widowed
Suicide history	Family history of suicide, history of suicide attempts
Intelligence	Relatively high intelligence quotient
Vocational history	Unemployed, early vocational difficulties, poor work functioning
Social support	Social isolation, limited external support
Substance-abuse history	Current or past substance abuse, especially alcohol
Depressive symptoms	Significant depressive symptoms or mood, depressive episode at last psychiatric visit, sense of hopelessness, hostility, depression, paranoid ideation, obsessive-compulsiveness, hospitalization for which a depressive episode was part of diagnosis
Psychotic symptoms	Command hallucinations, negative association with positive symptoms
Awareness of illness	Fear of further mental deterioration, awareness of deteriorative effects of schizophrenia
Course of illness	Frequent hospitalizations, recent discharge, acute exacerbations, worsening disease trend, frequent relapses and rehospitalizations, high post-discharge levels of psychopathology and functional impairment
Length of illness	Shorter duration of illness
Medication	Not receiving antipsychotics or relatively low or high antipsychotic doses

8

periods without its use. Clozapine may provide benefits by its ability to be used to treat TD, positive symptoms, and depressive symptoms without producing EPS. Additionally, there is extensive evidence that diminished serotoninergic activity may be related to suicide. Both animal and clinical studies have shown that a reduction in central serotonin function appears to be associated with suicidal, parasuicidal, and impulsive-aggressive behavior. The reduction of suicide risk in schizophrenic patients by clozapine is consistent with its reported antidepressant effects, which are achieved, in part, by normalization of serotoninergic function. The release of serotonin in the prefrontal cortex is seen with long-term clozapine therapy. The other SGADs have not yet been reported effective for decreasing suicide attempts. Risperidone, olanzapine, quetiapine, ziprasidone, and aripiprazole may be beneficial due to their lower side effect profiles and their effect on serotonin. Studies with these new agents are needed in this important area.

SUGGESTED READING

Brieden T, Ujeyl M, Naber D. Psychopharmacological treatment of aggression in schizophrenic patients. *Pharmacopsychiatry*. 2002;35:83-89.

Buckley PF. The role of typical and atypical antipsychotic medications in the management of agitation and aggression. *J Clin Psychiatry*. 1999;60(suppl 10):52-60.

Harkavy-Friedman JM, Nelson E. Management of the suicidal patient with schizophrenia. *Psychiatr Clin North Am*. 1997;20: 625-640.

Kane JM. Pharmacologic treatment of schizophrenia. *Biol Psychiatry*. 1999;46:1396-1408.

Meltzer HY. Suicide in schizophrenia: risk factors and clozapine treatment. *J Clin Psychiatry*. 1998;59(suppl 3):15-20.

Palmer DD, Henter ID, Wyatt RJ. Do antipsychotic medications decrease the risk of suicide in patients with schizophrenia? *J Clin Psychiatry*. 1999;60(suppl 2):100-103.

Radomsky ED, Haas GL, Mann JJ, Sweeney JA. Suicidal behavior in patients with schizophrenia and other psychotic disorders. *Am J Psychiatry*. 1999;156:1590-1595.

Schatzberg AF, De Battista C. Phenomenology and treatment of agitation. *J Clin Psychiatry*. 1999;60(suppl 15):17-20.

Steinert T, Wiebe C, Gebhardt RP. Aggressive behavior against self and others among first-admission patients with schizophrenia. *Psychiatr Serv*. 1999;50:85-90.

Volavka J, Citrome L. Atypical antipsychotics in the treatment of the persistently aggressive psychotic patient: methodological concerns. *Schizophr Res*. 1999;35(suppl):S23-S33.

8

9

Long-Acting Antipsychotic Drugs

Depot preparations of conventional antipsychotic medications were developed to aid with adherence to long-term drug therapy. The reported benefits of depot preparations include:
- Elimination of bioavailability problems
- Assurance of drug delivery
- A better strategy for low-dose therapy.

Disadvantages include:
- Potential for irreversible and unpleasant side effects
- Time required to reach optimal dosing
- Inability to immediately withdraw the drug if side effects develop
- Patients' feelings of being controlled.

Within state mental health facilities, 12% to 39% of all patients given traditional antipsychotics receive them in depot formulations. However, the overall use of depot medications in outpatient settings in the United States is low, representing only about 2% of all antipsychotic prescriptions. The best predictor of a person receiving a depot antipsychotic agent rather than an oral antipsychotic is a previous prescription for a depot antipsychotic. Younger patients, blacks, and Hispanics are more likely than whites and older patients to receive depot antipsychotics. Although clinicians widely believe that depot preparations increase patient adherence, there has been debate as to the extent to which long-acting injectable antipsychotics decrease relapse and rehospitalization rates when compared with oral agents. Long-acting second-generation antipsychotic drugs (SGADs) may provide great benefits in long-term adherence as compared with conventional depot agents.

Conventional Depot Agents

Depot preparations of two antipsychotics (fluphenazine decanoate and enanthate and haloperidol decanoate) are available in the United States. These are esterified antipsychotics formulated in sesame seed oil for deep intramuscular (IM) injection. Because these are long-acting preparations, patients should be exposed to the oral form of the drug prior to their first injection to minimize the possibility of long-acting side effects. With initial depot dosing, oral supplementation may temporarily be necessary. Care must be taken not to increase the depot preparation too rapidly, because steady state is only reached after four to five dosing intervals. Pain at the injection site is frequently reported with depot formulations and is a major cause of nonadherence.

The pharmacokinetics of the depot agents is a useful parameter for strategic dosing. Patients may be dosed with fluphenazine decanoate at a 1- to 3-week interval, while haloperidol decanoate is usually given once a month. There is much variability in dosing, however; conversion from an oral to a depot antipsychotic and maintenance dosing recommendations are shown in Table 9.1.

Based on the recommendations given in Table 9.1, a reasonable estimate is that fluphenazine decanoate 0.5 mL given every 2 weeks is equivalent to oral fluphenazine 10 mg/day. A maintenance dose of haloperidol decanoate 150 mg every 4 weeks is equivalent to oral haloperidol 10 mg/day. There remains great debate, however, as to the appropriate dosing and dosing interval of current conventional depot formulations.

TABLE 9.1 — MAINTENANCE DOSING RECOMMENDATIONS AND CONVERSION FROM ORAL TO DEPOT ANTIPSYCHOTIC DRUGS

Drug	Starting Dose	Maintenance Dose
Haloperidol decanoate	20 × oral haloperidol	10-15 oral haloperidol
	100-450 mg/28 d	50-300 mg/28 d
Fluphenazine decanoate	1.2 × oral fluphenazine	Based on starting dose and clinical response
	12.5-75 mg/7-21 d	
Fluphenazine enanthate	12.5-100 mg/ 7-21 d	Based on starting dose and clinical response

Some evidence suggests that similar efficacy is attained by giving injections at wider intervals (eg, every 6 weeks) to patients on a stable dose of antipsychotics. Also, based on several studies, fluphenazine decanoate may be associated with less relapse risk and lower rates of extrapyramidal symptoms (EPS) than haloperidol decanoate.

Second-Generation Depot Agents

A long-acting, injectable formulation of risperidone (Risperdal Consta) is the long-acting SGAD closest to being available in the United States. A new drug application has been filed and the Food and Drug Administration (FDA) has requested additional information. This drug formulation is gradually released into the body using a microsphere technology that maintains stable blood levels for 2 weeks. The active drug is contained in a saline-based solution rather than an oil-based one; only 2% of patients who received this formulation have complained of injection-site pain.

■ Pharmacology and Pharmacokinetics

Long-acting risperidone is an aqueous suspension containing risperidone in a matrix of glycolic acid–lactate copolymer. Gradual hydrolysis of the copolymer at the site of injection occurs over 2 weeks. A 2-week injection ensures the lowest fluctuation between peak and trough plasma levels. Therapeutic plasma levels are usually reached 3 to 4 weeks after starting the depot microspheres.

■ Dosing and Efficacy

Long-acting injectable risperidone should initially be given as a 25-, 50-, or 75-mg dose every 2 weeks (Table 9.2). Oral supplementation during the first 3 weeks is recommended (up to 4 mg/day) to ensure therapeutic plasma levels in the initial weeks. The IM injection should be administered in the gluteal area. Injectable dosing recommendations should be based on oral dosage, and all doses appear to have similar efficacy. Furthermore, studies reflect that efficacy is maintained for at least 1 year.

TABLE 9.2 — ORAL AND DEPOT DOSING RECOMMENDATIONS FOR RISPERIDONE	
Oral Dosing (mg/d)	**Depot Dosing (mg/2 wk)**
1-2	25
2-4	50
4-6	75

■ Adverse Effects

Extrapyramidal side effects were reported in 26% of patients in phase III clinical trials with no differences noted among dosing groups. Hyperkinesis accounted for one half of the reported cases, while dystonia was reported in less than 2% of patients. No patients dropped out of the studies due to EPS. The overall incidence of prolactin-related adverse events was approximately 6%, with a higher incidence in the 75-mg group than the 25- and 50-mg/day groups. Impotence occurred in about 2% of patients. Menstrual complaints, galactorrhea, and gynecomastia were all ≤1%. The most commonly occurring adverse effects are listed in Table 9.3.

TABLE 9.3 — MOST COMMON ADVERSE EFFECTS FOR LONG-ACTING RISPERIDONE IN PHASE III CLINICAL TRIALS			
Side Effect	**25 mg** **(_n_ = 120)**	**50 mg** **(_n_ = 228)**	**75 mg** **(_n_ = 267)**
Anxiety	16 (13%)	56 (25%)	77 (29%)
Psychosis	12 (10%)	22 (10%)	73 (27%)
Insomnia	16 (13%)	49 (22%)	65 (24%)
Depression	16 (13%)	28 (12%)	45 (17%)
Headache	10 (8%)	31 (14%)	33 (12%)
Fatigue	8 (7%)	21 (9%)	23 (9%)
Dizziness	5 (4%)	19 (8%)	19 (7%)

9

■ Studies

Studies thus far demonstrate the superior efficacy of risperidone injectable over placebo and the successful conversion from oral to depot risperidone without compromising efficacy and safety. While many data remain unpublished for long-acting risperidone, other data suggest that rehospitalization rates are <20% annually and that quality of life may be improved.

Other Long-Acting Formulations

A long-acting injectable form of olanzapine is currently in phase III trials and may be available in 2004. Iloperidone oral and long-acting injectable formulations are both currently in phase III trials.

Surgically implantable long-acting formulations containing haloperidol are in preclinical study. An implantable device capable of delivering antipsychotic medication for a period of 5 months is being developed. In contrast to depot formulations, implantable pellets could offer a degree of reversibility by removal of implants if unacceptable side effects occurred. The implants have been characterized for *in vitro* kinetics as well as *in vivo* bioactivity testing in rodents.

SUGGESTED READING

Barnes TR, Curson DA. Long-term depot antipsychotics. A risk-benefit assessment. *Drug Saf.* 1994;10:464-479.

Carpenter WT, Buchanan RW, Kirkpatrick B, Lann HD, Breier AF, Summerfelt AT. Comparative effectiveness of fluphenazine decanoate injections every 2 weeks versus every 6 weeks. *Am J Psychiatry*. 1999;156:412-418.

Gerlach J. Depot neuroleptics in relapse prevention: advantages and disadvantages. *Int Clin Psychopharmacol.* 1995;9(suppl 5):17-20.

Siegel SJ, Winey KI, Gur RE, et al. Surgically implantable long-term antipsychotic delivery systems for the treatment of schizophrenia. *Neuropsychopharmacology.* 2002;26:817-823.

Valenstein M, Copeland LA, Owen R, Blow FC, Visnic S. Adherence assessments and the use of depot antipsychotics in patients with schizophrenia. *J Clin Psychiatry.* 2001;62:545-551.

10 Continuation and Maintenance Therapy With Antipsychotic Drugs

Stabilization and Maintenance Therapy

If a patient has improved on a particular antipsychotic medication or medication regimen, the patient should continue to receive this same therapy at the same dose for the next 6 months before a lower maintenance dose is considered for continued treatment. Premature lowering of the dose or discontinuation of the medication during this phase may lead to relatively rapid relapse. Patients who have been stable for over 6 months and have no positive symptoms may be candidates for a dose reduction. This should be done gradually and to no less than at least one fifth of the usual maintenance dose as long as the patient remains stable.

Reviewing the need for maintenance antipsychotic medication should be done at least annually. Patients who have had no or very few symptoms throughout the year of maintenance treatment should be considered for a trial period without medication. Once this decision is made, the medication should be tapered slowly and gradually over many months. More frequent monitoring or visits are recommended and the use of early intervention strategies such as education about early relapse symptoms is important during this time. In patients who experience multiple episodes of symptoms, maintenance therapy should be continued for at least 5 years and probably indefinitely. The use of antipsychotics should continue in patients with suicidal or aggressive behavior. The long-term benefits of continuous antipsychotic medication are still not well understood because of the side effects and low adherence with conventional agents. Long-term studies of second-generation antipsychotic drugs (SGADs) suggest that benefits of these agents may accumulate over years of continued use.

Risperidone is the only SGAD with an approved indication from the Food and Drug Administration for the prevention of relapse. During long-term treatment, 60% of patients relapsed while taking haloperidol as compared with only 34% of those taking risperidone. Patients who were taking risperidone for 1 year also had greater reductions in the severity of psychotic symptoms and extrapyramidal symptoms (EPS) than those taking haloperidol. Aripiprazole and olanzapine have also been shown to be superior to haloperidol in long-term maintenance treatment by having a lower risk of relapse and less EPS. Relapse rates are lower with ziprasidone as compared to placebo, however, comparative studies with traditional antipsychotics are not available for ziprasidone or quetiapine.

Adherence

People with schizophrenia are often known to be noncompliant with medication. Factors that contribute to nonadherence with therapy include:

- Side effects
- Lack of insight
- Belief that the medication is ineffective.

Specific factors have predicted higher rates of nonadherence (Table 10.1). Older, grandiose, substance-abusing, and deficit patients have more difficulty with adherence. Adherence is difficult to quantify, measure, and study because adherence is rarely an all-or-none phenomenon, but may include mistakes in dosing, tim-

TABLE 10.1 — FACTORS RELATED TO COMPLIANCE

Patient-Related Factors
- Greater illness severity or grandiosity
- Lack of insight
- Substance-abuse comorbidity

Medication-Related Factors
- Dysphoric medication side effects
- Subtherapeutic or excessively high doses

Environmental Factors
- Inadequate support or supervision
- Practical barriers, such as lack of money or transportation

Clinician-Related Factors
- Poor therapeutic alliance

Adapted from: Fenton WS, et al. *Schizophr Bull.* 1997;23:637-651.

ing, omitting doses, or taking medications that are not prescribed. Estimates of nonadherence range from approximately 24% to 88%, with a mean of approximately 50% of people with schizophrenia who are nonadherent with prescribed therapy. Patients who are nonadherent have approximately a 4-fold greater risk of relapse than those who are compliant. Physicians often overestimate the adherence of their patients, which, in turn, does not allow them to consider nonadherence as a likely explanation for treatment failures.

Between 25% and 66% of patients who discontinue prescribed antipsychotic therapy cited adverse effects as the primary reason for nonadherence. Both self and physician ratings of side effects are associated with higher rates of nonadherence. EPS (most notably akathisia), sexual dysfunction, and weight gain are the adverse effects that lead to the greatest nonadherence. Second-generation antipsychotic drugs are associated with better rates of adherence, which is most likely attributable to better side effect profiles. This leads to lowering rates of relapse and rehospitalization, improving patient care, and reducing overall costs (see Chapter 15, *Outcomes and Health-Services Research*). A good relationship between the patient and the physician is important to establish rapport and trust, the groundwork for enhancing a patient's acceptance of the therapy. Patient and family education, including expectations and potential adverse effects, is important. The emergence of adverse events should be taken seriously and treated immediately.

SUGGESTED READING

Fenton WS, Blyler CR, Heinssen RK. Determinants of medication compliance in schizophrenia: empirical and clinical findings. *Schizophr Bull.* 1997;23:637-651.

Hogarty GE, Ulrich RF. The limitations of antipsychotic medication on schizophrenia relapse and adjustment and the contributions of psychosocial treatment. *J Psychiatr Res.* 1998;32:243-250.

Marder SR. Antipsychotic drugs and relapse prevention. *Schizophr Res.* 1999;35(suppl):S87-S92.

Robinson D, Woerner MG, Alvir JM, et al. Predictors of relapse following response from a first episode of schizophrenia or schizoaffective disorder. *Arch Gen Psychiatry.* 1999;56:241-247.

11 Treatment-Resistant Schizophrenia

One fifth to one third of all cases of schizophrenia are resistant to drug treatment. These patients are highly symptomatic and require extensive periods of hospital care. There has been a great deal of excitement following the demonstration of clozapine's efficacy in inpatients with treatment-resistant schizophrenia. However, clozapine treatment carries with it significant morbidity, including:

- Serious side effects
- Need for ongoing weekly blood monitoring
- High cost.

Many clinicians and patients hoped that other new antipsychotics would share clozapine's effectiveness without its most serious side effects. However, no other antipsychotic has clozapine's efficacy in this patient group. The incidence of resistance to antipsychotic therapy and thus the need for clozapine in such patients is lessened by optimal use of second-generation and depot antipsychotics.

Chronicity vs Treatment Resistance

Commonly, treatment resistance has been considered to be roughly equivalent to chronic or frequent hospitalization. This is not an adequate definition. Patients should also have current and persistent positive symptoms of psychosis and at least moderate overall severity of illness in order for nonresponsiveness to apply, as chronic hospitalization can occur despite low levels of symptoms.

Many people with schizophrenia who have been chronically hospitalized may not be truly resistant to drug treatment. Inadequate psychosocial programming, poor adherence to prescribed drug therapy, and a history of committing violence are all risk factors for chronic hospitalization. Therefore, an optimized medication and treatment trial should be employed before a patient's illness is considered nonresponsive. In addition, both the effects of drug nonadherence and extrapyramidal symptoms (EPS) can mimic true treatment resistance. At least a 1- to 2-year course of persistent symptoms should be considered one of the criteria for treatment resistance in schizophrenia because of the waxing and waning course of this illness.

Definition of Treatment Resistance

The most accepted current criteria for treatment resistance in schizophrenia were first widely used by Kane and associates. These criteria, modified for clinical use, are presented in Table 11.1.

Defining Adequate Drug Trials

Two retrospective drug trial failures are as effective as three in screening for treatment resistance. People not responsive to two adequate antipsychotic trials (one retrospective and one prospective) have less than a 7% chance of responding to another trial. The Food and Drug Administration (FDA) guidelines for clozapine's use, as reflected in the product labeling for Clozaril, also state that people should fail to respond to two separate trials of antipsychotics before being treated with clozapine.

It is generally recognized that a 4- to 6-week period (rather than strictly a 6-week period) is adequate for a treatment trial of an antipsychotic. Doses ≥400 mg/day of chlorpromazine have been shown to be ad-

**TABLE 11.1 — CRITERIA FOR TREATMENT
RESISTANCE IN SCHIZOPHRENIA**

- Persistent positive psychotic symptoms of at least two of four common positive symptoms:
  - Hallucinatory behavior
  - Suspiciousness
  - Unusual thought content
  - Conceptual disorganization
- Current presence of at least a moderately severe illness
- Persistence of illness: no period of good social and/or occupational functioning within the past 5 years
- Drug-refractory condition defined as at least two periods of treatment within the preceding 5 years with appropriate doses of conventional or second-generation antipsychotics, each without clinically significant symptom relief

equate to block 80% to 90% of dopamine receptors (thought to be the target of this drug action). Higher doses produce no direct therapeutic benefit, even in patients not responsive to therapy, and do not have greater efficacy than lower doses in acute treatment. Therefore, two 4- to 6-week trials of 400 to 600 mg chlorpromazine are now accepted as a standard for an adequate trial.

Neurobiology of Treatment Resistance in Schizophrenia

Until the arrival of standardized criteria for defining treatment resistance, research into the neurobiologic nature of the problem had been scant. Recently, however, with the use of more objective criteria, some consistent findings have been seen. There is a relative paucity of data in this area, and more research needs to be done. People with treatment-resistant schizophrenia appear to have increased cortical atrophy on magnetic resonance imaging (MRI) compared with those with responsive illness. This is particularly true if they have predominant negative symptoms.

Lack of response to early treatment is also predictive of nonresponse. The most intriguing finding about predicting which new drugs may be effective in treatment-resistant schizophrenia has been the fact that such people appear to have lower catecholamine levels in the cerebrospinal fluid (CSF). Clozapine response has been associated with low ratios of CSF homovanillic acid to 5-hydroxyindoleacetic acid. These findings suggest that drugs with low dopamine antagonism and high serotoninergic antagonism may be particularly useful in treatment-resistant schizophrenia.

Drug Therapy for Treatment Resistance

Historically, drug therapy for treatment-resistant schizophrenia centered either on the use of different dose strategies of conventional antipsychotics or on the use of adjunct agents such as lithium, β-blocking drugs, anticonvulsants, and benzodiazepines. Since the arrival of clozapine, attention in the field has shifted to a greater focus on the use of new antipsychotics for treatment resistance in schizophrenia. This interest has occurred because of the demonstration of the superior efficacy of clozapine and the fact that new antipsychotics must have been shown to have either significantly fewer side effects or improved efficacy compared with a conventional antipsychotic (usually haloperidol) in order to be marketed in the United States.

Conventional Antipsychotic Drugs

Conventional antipsychotic drugs have long been the first-line drug therapy for treating schizophrenia. In controlled trials of people with drug-resistant symptoms, fewer than 5% responded after having their drug therapy changed from one conventional antipsychotic to another. If no clinical improvement is seen after 2 weeks of therapy, adherence with medication should be evaluated. If the patient is adherent, a different drug trial should be considered after 4 to 6 weeks of minimal response.

Second-Generation Antipsychotic Drugs

Second-generation antipsychotic drugs should be the first consideration after the failure of conventional drug therapy. These drugs are also effective as first-line therapy (with the exception of clozapine, because of its serious side effects).

■ Clozapine

Clozapine was approved for use by the FDA in 1990 specifically for the treatment of patients whose symptoms do not adequately respond to conventional antipsychotic therapy, either because therapy was not effective or because it could not be continued secondary to intolerable side effects. It is still the only drug with proven efficacy in rigorously defined treatment-resistant schizophrenia, and approximately 30% of treatment-refractory patients will respond to this medication. However, fewer than 8% of new antipsychotic prescriptions are written for clozapine. This phenomenon of relative underusage probably relates to the cost and complexity of clozapine therapy. These arise from the need for long-term hematologic monitoring for agranulocytosis and persistent serious side effects, such as weight gain, sialorrhea, and sedation, that can accompany therapy with clozapine.

The optimal dose strategy for clozapine is a slow dose escalation. Patients should be evaluated for response at dose plateaus of 200 to 400 mg/day and 500 to 600 mg/day. Only patients with few side effects from clozapine should be titrated to doses higher than 600 mg/day. Patients should not be titrated to a higher dose of clozapine if myoclonus is present, since this side effect may precede the development of seizures.

■ **Risperidone**

It is been widely recognized that risperidone treatment is usually not effective in clozapine responders who are treatment-resistant. Risperidone is more effective than conventional antipsychotics for positive and affective symptoms in patients with acute schizophrenia. Wirshing and others found a 24% response rate to risperidone as compared with an 11% response rate to haloperidol after 4 weeks in patients who were treatment-resistant. Although risperidone does not appear to be as effective as clozapine for treatment resistance, it may be worth a trial even after traditional antipsychotics have failed prior to using clozapine.

■ **Olanzapine**

Olanzapine is effective in treatment-responsive schizophrenia, with superiority in negative and affective symptoms in acute patients. It has a low incidence of EPS and is not different from placebo in its incidence of akathisia. It does not, however, have clozapine-like efficacy in well-characterized treatment resistance. Conley and others found only a 7% response rate in a treatment-refractory population. Additionally, 40% of those treatment failures went on to respond to clozapine. Adequate clinical trial data for olanzapine are lacking; there does not appear to be any additional benefit at higher doses than those included in the package labeling.

■ Quetiapine

Quetiapine has been shown to be effective in treatment-responsive schizophrenia. There was no difference between placebo and quetiapine in the amount of EPS or akathisia in published trials to date. This drug is not more effective than haloperidol in acute schizophrenia. Quetiapine may also be an option before proceeding to clozapine treatment. Higher response rates were noted with quetiapine as compared with haloperidol. Higher dosing of quetiapine may be needed ($\geq$600 mg).

■ Ziprasidone and Aripiprazole

To date, little data are available on the use of ziprasidone and aripiprazole in patients with treatment-resistant schizophrenia. In chronic patients, aripiprazole was more effective than placebo; however, comparisons with other antipsychotics are not yet available.

Alternate Therapies

If patients remain refractory to treatment after trials of novel agents, alternate therapies should be considered, such as adjunct medication or electroconvulsive therapy (ECT). The data concerning the efficacy of these therapies are limited, but they may be of use in some patients.

■ Lithium and Anticonvulsants

Adjunct lithium therapy has been seen to be beneficial in some patients with treatment-resistant schizophrenia; however, these patients were often not defined by the rigorous criteria of later studies. These published trials of adjunct lithium, which are positive, have been conducted with small numbers of patients, and often the criteria for defining treatment resistance were not clear or were overinclusive. More recent reports have found no benefits with adjunct lithium therapy and fluphenazine decanoate. Lithium should be used with caution in combination with conventional antipsychotics or clozapine because of the recognized dangers of delirium, encephalopathy, and neurotoxicity that have been reported with these combinations.

Carbamazepine and valproic acid have been observed to be effective in bipolar affective disorder and are often considered as adjunct therapy in patients with schizophrenia. However, trials involving these agents have had relatively few subjects. Positive effects seen with carbamazepine and valproate have been modest and usually involved nonspecific improvement in areas such as behavior and social adjustment. Carbamazepine should be used with caution due to reports of disorientation and ataxia associated with its use. It can also reduce the blood level of haloperidol by as much as 50%. Carbamazepine should not be used in combination with clozapine. There are few data on newer anticonvulsants, although positive results have been noted with lamotrigine adjunctive treatment with clozapine. The addition of lamotrigine to other SGADs has not produced favorable results. Topiramate does not appear to increase efficacy of antipsychotic drugs.

■ Benzodiazepines

There have been several reports on the use of adjunct benzodiazepines in treatment-resistant schizophrenia. Results have been mixed, with some double-blind studies showing a treatment effect, while other studies are negative. Given that patients with schizophrenia frequently experience anxiety and irritability, it is not surprising that benzodiazepines often prove to be useful agents in the treatment of this disorder.

There is no firm evidence for a specific adjunct anti-psychotic effect with these agents, however. They should be used with caution because of the risks of chronic sedation, fatigue ataxia, and dependence. There are some reports of behavioral disinhibition with these drugs and the possibility of synergistic respiratory toxicity with clozapine.

■ Other Therapies

There are historical studies suggesting that β-blockers and reserpine may be useful in refractory schizophrenia. However, there are no available controlled studies with current diagnostic criteria. There is limited evidence that long-term therapy with either of these strategies is beneficial. There have been no controlled studies of ECT to date in treatment-resistant schizophrenic patients. Before the use of clozapine, there was some evidence from uncontrolled trials that ECT provided benefit for treatment-resistant patients, but usually the effect of ECT has been the most robust in patients with an illness of short duration. There have been a few open trials of ECT in patients who had an inadequate clozapine response. These trials showed some benefit from ECT. However, issues of persistence of effect and long-term maintenance of these patients have not yet been addressed.

There are very few positive data available supporting the use of two antipsychotic medications. The introduction of another antipsychotic should only occur when optimization of all other treatments has failed. The concurrent use should be objectively rated for improvements in symptoms. If no significant improvements are seen, the second agent should be discontinued, since the risk for adverse effects outweighs the benefits. The most favorable concomitant data are for risperidone augmentation of clozapine.

Summary

A defined approach to patients with treatment-resistant schizophrenia is critical. The practices outlined in Table 11.2 should maximize the likelihood of a successful outcome for an antipsychotic drug trial for treatment resistance.

Since the antipsychotics being introduced today may have different mechanisms of action than conventional antipsychotics and than each other, clinicians will need to explore the possibility of response who have each of these new agents in turn with their patients with persistently refractory symptoms. To date, clozapine is the only medication with demonstrated efficacy in treatment resistance. The differential efficacy of new drugs in treatment-resistant schizophrenia will only be clear when well-designed double-blind studies using rigorous entry criteria are completed.

SUGGESTED READING

Bustillo JR, Lauriello J, Keith SJ. Schizophrenia: improving outcome. *Harv Rev Psychiatry.* 1999;6:229-240.

Conley RR, Buchanan RW. Evaluation of treatment-resistant schizophrenia. *Schizophr Bull.* 1997;23:663-674.

Kane J, Honigfeld G, Singer J, Meltzer H. Clozapine for the treatment-resistant schizophrenia. A double-blind comparison with chlorpromazine. *Arch Gen Psychiatry.* 1988;45:789-796.

Kane JM. Treatment-resistant schizophrenic patients. *J Clin Psychiatry.* 1996;57(suppl 9):35-40.

Sheitman BB, Lieberman JA. The natural history and pathophysiology of treatment resistant schizophrenia. *J Psychiatr Res.* 1998; 32:143-150.

Wahlbeck K, Cheine M, Essali A, Adams C. Evidence of clozapine's effectiveness in schizophrenia: a systematic review and meta-analysis of randomized trials. *Am J Psychiatry.* 1999;156: 990-999.

Wirshing DA, Marshall BD Jr, Green MF, Mintz J, Marder SR, Wirshing WC. Risperidone in treatment-refractory schizophrenia. *Am J Psychiatry.* 1999;156:1374-1379.

11

TABLE 11.2 — APPROACH TO PATIENTS WITH TREATMENT-RESISTANT SCHIZOPHRENIA

- Identification of defined target symptoms. Antipsychotics are most helpful for the positive symptoms of psychosis: hallucinations, delusions, and thought disorder. Newer medications may also be helpful in reducing negative symptoms, such as poor socialization, withdrawal, and affective blunting, particularly if these are secondary to extrapyramidal symptoms of conventional antipsychotics. Clozapine has been shown to be effective in hostile, aggressive, psychotic patients. Understanding the target symptoms for a specific drug trial will allow for greater clarity in defining the parameters of success and failure.

- The systematic use of drugs at sufficient dosages and for a sufficient duration to establish efficacy. This is particularly critical before adjunct drugs are used since they may complicate the therapeutic situation to the point where defining the optimal drug treatment for a patient is not possible.

- Consideration that medication intolerance, noncompliance, inadequate social support, and inadequate psychosocial treatment may create the appearance of treatment resistance. A consideration of these factors should precede the declaration that any drug therapy is a failure. Although therapeutic ranges of most antipsychotics are not well established, measuring blood levels may be useful to establish compliance and to rule out the unlikely event of poor medication absorption.

- Exhausting the utility of single agents before using multiple agents. There is tremendous pressure for the clinician to find a drug to rapidly treat every psychological problem manifest in a patient. It is important to remember that no adjunct agent has ever been shown to robustly improve antipsychotic response. Hostility, irritability, insomnia, and withdrawal can all be secondary to psychosis and may resolve only after a patient has experienced a good antipsychotic drug effect.

- Aggressively preventing extrapyramidal symptoms through the appropriate choice of primary therapy. With the arrival of antipsychotic agents that are clearly effective at doses that do not produce extrapyramidal symptoms in the vast majority of patients, we should be able to almost eliminate persistent side effects as a reason for therapeutic failure.
- Maintaining a positive therapeutic attitude. There are more choices now for antipsychotic therapy than ever before, with new drugs appearing annually. Patients should be encouraged to think that there is good reason to be optimistic that some therapy will be found that will be beneficial to them, even if they have a history of severe illness.

12 Antipsychotics in Special Populations

Treatment of Schizophrenia in Adolescents

The diagnosis of schizophrenia in children and adolescents is often difficult to make and should be differentiated from pervasive developmental disorders, attention-deficit/hyperactivity disorder, and language or communication disorders. If a child has prominent hallucinations or delusions, however, the diagnosis of schizophrenia should be considered. Onset before the age of 18 is often classified as early-onset schizophrenia, and those presenting with symptoms before the age of 14 are labeled patients with very-early-onset schizophrenia (VEOS). Although more male adolescents may develop VEOS than females (2:1), the overall prevalence is rare: 1/10,000 individuals. Auditory hallucinations are common and occur in approximately 80% of children and adolescents with schizophrenia. Command hallucinations are the most frequently occurring type of hallucination. The content and context of hallucinations in children and adolescents vary by age, with younger children tending to be less complex and less "fixed." Childhood themes, such as monsters or animals, are common but should not be mistaken for normal childhood imagination and imaginary images.

Treatment of psychotic children and adolescents ideally involves an intensive and comprehensive program. A highly structured environment with special education and psychoeducation is recommended. Day treatment, hospitalization, or long-term residential treatment may be necessary. Pharmacologic treatment is indicated if positive psychotic symptoms cause significant impairments or interfere with other interventions. Conventional antipsychotics have modest efficacy in children and adolescents (expressed in chlorpromazine [CPZ] equivalent dosages) at doses between 10 CPZ to 200 CPZ equivalents. Younger patients appear to be less responsive to pharmacotherapy than adults, however.

The low-potency agents should be avoided in this population because of sedation and cognitive dulling, which may interfere with school work. Adolescents are more vulnerable to extrapyramidal symptoms (EPS), namely dystonic reactions, than are adults. Due to concerns with EPS and tardive dyskinesia (TD) in this group, many children and adolescents are being given second-generation antipsychotic drugs (SGADs). A few open trials have reported on the use of clozapine in children and adolescents. Although most patients experience improvement during clozapine therapy, side effects in this population may be more pronounced than in adults. The most prominent symptoms seen are:

- Somnolence
- Hypersalivation
- Weight gain.

Children and adolescents tend on average to gain more weight than reported in the adult literature. Mean weight gains are over 15 lb in 6 weeks with conventional antipsychotics. The risk for agranulocytosis appears to be similar to the risk in adults. Children and adolescents who have been found to be resistant to at least two trials of antipsychotics including another SGAD may benefit from a trial of clozapine. They should be treated initially with lower doses than adult patients and be titrated at a slower rate. Side effects should be monitored closely during initiation and throughout maintenance therapy. Enuresis may occur with clozapine therapy and often at higher rates in children and adolescents than in adults.

The use of risperidone, quetiapine, and olanzapine has also been reported in open studies and case report series. These medications appear to be similar in regard to efficacy in this population, and side effects are similar to those observed in the adult population. Weight gain with these agents, as well, is more pronounced than in the adult population. Of these agents, olanzapine causes the greatest amount of weight gain. Prolactin-related adverse effects, especially galactorrhea, menstrual changes, and gynecomastia, occur more frequently in the younger population than in adults. Risperidone causes some of these problems more frequently than the other SGADs, but they are generally dose related.

Initial dosing for risperidone in children and adolescents should be 0.25 to 0.5 mg qd or bid. The range for treatment is between 0.5 and 5 mg/day. Olanzapine should be initiated at 5 mg/day and titrated to 10 to 20 mg/day. Quetiapine doses are between 200 and 800 mg/day. Few data are available for ziprasidone and aripiprazole. Children metabolize these drugs more rapidly than do adults but also require lower plasma levels for efficacy. Informed consent, the rationale for treatment, and potential risks and benefits of therapy **12** should be addressed with the parents/guardians prior to treatment with any antipsychotic medication, and assent should be obtained from the child. Standardized clinician ratings, such as the Positive and Negative Syndrome Scales derived from the Children's Psychiatric Rating Scale, are sensitive to antipsychotic improvement in children and adolescents.

Treatment of Psychosis in the Elderly

In the elderly, the prevalence of various types of depression, anxiety, dementia, and psychotic disorders can be as high as 50% for nursing home residents. In fact, for institutionalized patients, antipsychotics are the most widely prescribed psychotropic drugs. Because of the widespread and unnecessary use of these agents in this population in the past, Congress passed regulations for their use in 1987. This led to the introduction of the Omnibus Budget Reconciliation Act and the Nursing Home Reform Amendments through the Health Care Financing Administration. These regulations set specific standards for allowable dosages and indications for psychotropic drugs in regular use and on an as-needed basis.

Antipsychotics can be safe and effective for the treatment of psychosis if used at lower doses than commonly used in young adults. Older adults are particularly vulnerable to side effects of conventional antipsychotics. Parkinsonian symptoms reportedly occur in >50% of all elderly patients receiving these agents, and the cumulative annual incidence of TD in middle-aged and elderly patients is >25%. The likelihood of reversing this potentially debilitating condition diminishes with age. Other adverse effects of these agents that are often intolerable in the older population include orthostatic hypotension and anticholinergic effects. Orthostasis is estimated to occur in 5% to 30% of geriatric patients and is a major contributing factor in the occurrence of falls. The elderly are more prone to consequences associated with falls, such as bone fractures, injuries, and resulting dependency. Low-potency agents and clozapine are more likely to cause significant drops in orthostatic blood pressure. Anticholinergic agents in the elderly may cause such side effects as:

- Constipation
- Dry mouth
- Urinary retention
- Cognitive impairment.

The elderly are especially sensitive to these effects, and the use of laxatives or stool softeners is particularly high in nursing homes. Cognitive impairment may lead to decreased independence, and a more rapid decline in cognitive functioning may occur in elderly patients treated with antipsychotics than in the younger adult population.

Clozapine has been used successfully in the elderly population at lower doses than in younger adult patients. Mean doses have ranged from 50 to 300 mg/day, with a much slower rate of titration. Clozapine may be a good selection for treating psychotic elderly patients with preexisting parkinsonism because of this drug's lower affinity for dopamine $(D)_2$ receptors in the striatum. Clinically, however, it is a poorly tolerated antipsychotic in geriatric patients and should be used with caution. The risk for agranulocytosis appears to be about 4% in the elderly population, with older women being at highest risk. The risk for seizure activity is increased in the elderly, and sedation is one of the major reasons for discontinuation. Clozapine therapy should be initiated at 12.5 to 25 mg/day given in two divided doses, titrating by increments of 12.5 mg over 5 to 7 days.

Risperidone has been shown to be effective in the elderly with schizophrenia, schizoaffective disorder, major depression with psychotic features, bipolar disorder, and delusional disorder. A dose range of 0.5 to 3 mg is the optimal range for the treatment of psychotic symptoms in the elderly. Initially, patients should receive 0.25 to 0.5 mg taken once daily, with titration in increments not greater than 0.5 mg/24 hours. In most studies, risperidone has been well tolerated, with the most common side effects being hypotension, orthostasis, sedation, and EPS. Olanzapine and quetiapine have been reported to be of benefit in the elderly population. Ziprasidone should be used with

12

caution due to its propensity to prolong the QTc interval. Aripiprazole appears to be effective and well tolerated in the elderly. A starting dose of olanzapine should be 2.5 to 10 mg/day and increased by 5 mg no more frequently than every 7 days to a target range of 10 to 20 mg/day. Lower doses of quetiapine should be used as well. These agents appear to have adverse-effect profiles similar to those in the adult population. Quetiapine may be the best selection for psychosis associated with Parkinson's disease. More data are needed for the newer antipsychotic drugs to confirm relative safety and efficacy of these medications in this population.

Treatment of Schizophrenia in Dually Diagnosed Patients

The prevalence of substance abuse among persons with schizophrenia is significantly higher than in the general population. Conservative estimates are that one third to as many as one half of people with schizophrenia abuse alcohol and illicit drugs. Dually diagnosed patients are more likely to be nonadherent to treatment and medications often because of side effects. These people also have a poorer response rate to conventional antipsychotics and have higher rates of rehospitalization. For patients discharged on conventional antipsychotics, substance abuse is one of the most significant reasons for readmission. EPS may occur more frequently in patients who are substance abusing, and abusing drugs and alcohol is a risk factor for developing TD.

There is evidence that substance-abusing patients respond differently to conventional antipsychotics compared with non–substance-abusing patients. A few studies have reported that substance-abusing patients receiving fixed doses of haloperidol and perphenazine had a poorer response and more readmissions than non–substance-abusing patients. This is likely due to the fact that substance abusers suffer increased rates of parkinsonian side effects from conventional antipsychotics and are less adherent than nonabusing patients. Substance abuse itself can lead to chronic psychosis and psychotic relapse. Despite the fact that substance-abusing patients do poorly with conventional antipsychotic treatment, this group has been found to have better premorbid functioning and less functional impairment than non–substance-abusing schizophrenic patients. It is possible that while patients in this group are difficult to treat, they may also present a subgroup with a better potential for recovery and perhaps a better opportunity for successful reintegration into community living.

Second-generation antipsychotic drugs may offer effective clinical treatment for schizophrenic patients involved in comorbid substance abuse. It has been reported that treatment with clozapine and olanzapine is associated with similar response rates between patients with and without substance-abuse histories. Additionally, these medications are associated with better adherence rates than conventional agents, as well as lower rates of rehospitalization. Further evidence indicates that clozapine treatment may actually be associated with a reduction in the use of drugs and alcohol. Case reports of patients treated with risperidone who are substance abusers reveal that it not only is efficacious for symptoms but may help curb use as well. Thus substance-abusing patients may benefit from SGADs in terms of both better efficacy and adverse-effect profiles.

Treatment of Schizophrenia With Mood and Anxiety Symptoms

When Kraepelin first described psychosis, he divided symptoms into dementia praecox and manic-depressive psychosis. This division failed, however, to include many patients with mixed features. Approximately 30% to 60% of patients with schizophrenia report an episode of major depression at some point in their lifetime. Schizoaffective disorder or schizophrenia with concurrent depression is an example of patients with primary psychosis in conjunction with prominent mood symptoms. Although mood stabilizers and antidepressants are ineffective for psychosis, they may offer benefits to patients for relief of symptoms associated with mood. It is important to remember that as other medications are added to the regimen, specific target symptoms should be identified and objective rating criteria should be utilized to assess efficacy.

Second-generation antipsychotic drugs may be effective as monotherapy for schizoaffective disorder. Clozapine has been found to be more effective in patients with schizoaffective disorder than in those with schizophrenia. Schizoaffective disorder, in fact, has been found to be a predictor of clozapine response in treatment-resistant populations. There is accumulating evidence that risperidone, olanzapine, and quetiapine all may be beneficial for schizoaffective disorder as well as bipolar disorder. This evidence suggests that SGADs are more effective than conventional antipsychotics for mood symptoms. Monotherapy should be attempted in these disorders prior to polytherapy.

Anticonvulsants and mood stabilizers in combination with antipsychotics have been more effective for schizoaffective disorder than antipsychotics plus placebo. This has not been found to be true, however, for patients with schizophrenia lacking a mood component. Lithium, valproate, and carbamazepine appear to offer benefits, but few large well-controlled studies have looked at treatment specifically for schizoaffective disorder. Carbamazepine is a potent inducer of the cytochrome P450 (CYP450) 3A3/4 pathway, thus it potentially may lower blood levels of quetiapine. Carbamazepine should not be used concurrently with clozapine due to the risk for the occurrence of agranulocytosis. Lithium may increase leukocytes and thus has the potential to mask neutropenia with clozapine treatment. Valproate may increase plasma levels of clozapine or olanzapine through inhibition of CYP450 2D6. This is not a potent effect of valproate, but a few patients will experience an increase in plasma concentrations. Valproate and lithium also increase the risk for weight gain with antipsychotic treatment.

Little work has been done in looking at antidepressant use in combination with antipsychotics for the treatment of schizoaffective disorder or schizophrenia with depression. The most widely accepted data for patient depression with schizophrenia or schizoaffective disorder concern the treatment of depressive symptoms after stabilization of psychosis. If antidepressants are concurrently used, the possibility for drug interaction exists. Fluvoxamine, a potent inhibitor of the CYP450 1A2 isoenzyme, will increase blood levels of clozapine and olanzapine. Fluoxetine, paroxetine, and higher doses of sertraline may increase blood levels as well. SGADs, although not studied in monotherapy for depression, appear to intrinsically offer some benefits for affective symptoms such as anxiety and depression.

Patients who continue to exhibit significant symptoms of anxiety once stabilization of psychosis is accomplished may benefit from anxiolytic therapy. The concurrent use of benzodiazepines and clozapine should be avoided, if possible, due to the increased risk for sudden respiratory depression that may occur with the combination. Also, benzodiazepines may lead to cognitive dulling or paradoxic agitation. Thus in patients with deficits in cognitive functioning intrinsic to schizophrenia itself, the use of another contributing agent should be strongly evaluated. Buspirone may work for anxiety but may be less effective in patients who have already received benzodiazepine therapy.

SUGGESTED READING

Buckley PF. Substance abuse in schizophrenia: a review. *J Clin Psychiatry*. 1998;59(suppl 3):26-30.

Campbell M, Rapoport JL, Simpson GM. Antipsychotics in children and adolescents. *J Am Acad Child Adolesc Psychiatry*. 1999; 38:537-545.

Collaborative Working Group on Clinical Trial Evaluations. Treatment of special populations with the atypical antipsychotics. *J Clin Psychiatry*. 1998;59(suppl 12):46-52.

Findling RL, Schulz SC, Reed MD, Blumer JL. The antipsychotics. A pediatric perspective. *Pediatr Clin North Am*. 1998;45: 1205-1232.

Jeste DV, Rockwell E, Harris MJ, Lohr JB, Lacro J. Conventional vs newer antipsychotics in elderly patients. *Am J Geriatr Psychiatry*. 1999;7:70-76.

Krystal JH, D'Souza DC, Madonick S, Petrakis IL. Toward a rational pharmacotherapy of comorbid substance abuse in schizophrenic patients. *Schizophr Res*. 1999;35(suppl):S35-S49.

Levinson DF, Umapathy C, Musthaq M. Treatment of schizoaffective disorder and schizophrenia with mood symptoms. *Am J Psychiatry*. 1999;156:1138-1148.

Maixner SM, Mellow AM, Tandon R. The efficacy, safety, and tolerability of antipsychotics in the elderly. *J Clin Psychiatry*. 1999;60(suppl 8):29-41.

McClellan J, Werry JS. Practice parameters for the assessment and treatment of children and adolescents with schizophrenia. American Academy of Child and Adolescent Psychiatry. *J Am Acad Child Adolesc Psychiatry*. 1997;36(suppl 10):177S-193S.

Toren P, Laor N, Weizman A. Use of atypical neuroleptics in child and adolescent psychiatry. *J Clin Psychiatry*. 1998;59:644-656.

13 Drug Interactions With Antipsychotic Drugs

Pharmacokinetics is the study of how the body acts upon drugs, especially in terms of absorption, distribution, metabolism, and excretion. Interactions may occur during any of these processes as a drug is transported to and from its site of action and may result in a change in the plasma level or tissue distribution of the drug. Pharmacodynamics refers to the effect of the drugs on the body. This type of interaction occurs at biologically active receptor sites and results in a change in the pharmacologic effects of a given plasma level of the drug. This chapter will focus mainly on pharmacokinetic drug interactions.

Absorption

Gastrointestinal drug absorption can be altered by the concomitant administration of a second drug, food product, herbal supplement, or an environmental product that physically or chemically binds to the drug, increases or decreases gut motility, alters intestinal bacterial flora, or changes gastric pH. Antacids, charcoal, and cholestyramine are agents that can bind to other agents and form insoluble complexes. Antacids should always be given 2 hours apart from antipsychotics to avoid decreasing absorption. Most of the antipsychotic drugs are not affected by food. Absorption of quetiapine, however, may be increased with meals. Absorption is increased by approximately 60% to 70% when ziprasidone is given with meals. In addition, antipsychotic solutions should not be given with other solutions (such as carbamazepine and lithium) since insoluble complexes may form.

Distribution

In general, the antipsychotics have a relatively high affinity for plasma proteins, with most being >80% protein bound. A reversible equilibrium exists between bound and unbound drug; the unbound fraction is pharmacologically active, whereas the bound fraction is inactive and cannot be metabolized or excreted. When two drugs exist simultaneously in the plasma, competition for protein-binding sites may occur. This may result in the displacement of a previously bound drug, which, in the free state, becomes pharmacologically active. Interactions that occur by this mechanism are called "protein-binding interactions." Most protein-binding interactions are transient and are not clinically significant because the plasma-concentration change of free drug is generally quite small. Clinically significant interactions may occur with antipsychotics when given with another highly protein-bound drug with a low therapeutic index such as warfarin or phenytoin.

Metabolism

All antipsychotic agents are metabolized by hepatic microsomal enzymes to water-soluble compounds that can be excreted by the kidneys. The most important of the microsomal enzymes are the cytochrome P450 (CYP450) enzymes, a group of nonspecific mixed-function oxidases that play a major role in oxidative drug metabolism. Ziprasidone, however, is mostly metabolized by aldehyde oxidase. Although >30 isoenzymes have been identified in humans, three play major roles in the metabolism of antipsychotic medications:

- CYP450 2D6
- CYP450 1A2
- CYP450 3A3/4.

Not all individuals have the same CYP450 enzymes. If mutations occur in >1% of a specific population, it is termed pharmacogenetic polymorphism. For example, about 5% to 10% of whites are poor metabolizers via the CYP450 2D6 enzyme. Thus these people must metabolize drugs by alternative routes that may not be as efficient as the 2D6 route, leading to increases in plasma concentrations for the drug to be metabolized. The major enzymes for metabolism of second-generation antipsychotic drugs (SGADs) and a few known for traditional antipsychotics are listed in Table 13.1.

Other medications, food products, herbal supplements, and environmental factors may inhibit or induce any of these pathways, possibly lowering or raising plasma concentrations of any of the antipsychotic medications. Table 13.2 provides a list of some substances that may affect metabolism.

TABLE 13.1 — MAJOR ENZYMES FOR METABOLISM OF ANTIPSYCHOTIC DRUGS

Drug	Major Metabolic Pathway	Other Metabolic Pathways
Aripiprazole	3A4/2D6	—
Clozapine	1A2	3A3/4, 2D6
Haloperidol	2D6	—
Olanzapine	1A2	2D6
Perphenazine	2D6	—
Quetiapine	3A3/4	—
Risperidone	2D6	—
Thioridazine	2D6	—
Ziprasidone	3A3/4, aldehyde oxidase	—

13

TABLE 13.2 — SUBSTANCES THAT MAY AFFECT METABOLISM OF ANTIPSYCHOTIC DRUGS

Type of Agent	CYP450 1A2	CYP450 2D6	CYP450 3A3/4
Inducing agents	Cigarette smoking Omeprazole	—	Carbamazepine Phenytoin Phenobarbital Rifampin
Inhibiting agents	Fluvoxamine Fluoxetine (weak) Fluoroquinolines Cimetidine	Fluoxetine Paroxetine Sertraline (weak, dose-related) Tertiary tricyclic antidepressants Haloperidol (weak) Thioridazine (weak) Perphenazine (weak) Quinidine	Fluoxetine Nefazodone Ketoconazole Itraconazole Erythromycin Protease inhibitors Cisapride Verapamil Diltiazem Grapefruit

Abbreviations: CYP450, cytochrome P450.

A listing of likely interactions with SGADs that may be clinically significant appears in Table 13.3. Clinically meaningful interactions with risperidone and quetiapine are unlikely. Clozapine and olanzapine may be affected by other substances, and high blood levels of ziprasidone may lead to possible prolongations of the QT interval.

TABLE 13.3 — CLINICALLY IMPORTANT INTERACTIONS WITH SECOND-GENERATION ANTIPSYCHOTIC DRUGS

Drug	Drug Interaction
Clozapine	Inhibitors of cytochrome P450 (CYP450) 1A2 (fluvoxamine, others) can raise clozapine levels. Cigarette smoking can decrease clozapine level; watch for relapse if patient begins or increases smoking. Inhibitors of CYP450 2D6 can raise clozapine levels. Strong inhibitors of CYP450 3A3/4 can raise clozapine levels.
Olanzapine	Inhibitors of CYP450 1A2 can raise olanzapine levels. Cigarette smoking can decrease olanzapine levels. Inhibitors of CYP450 2D6 may raise olanzapine levels. Women have higher plasma concentrations than men; may need lower doses.
Ziprasidone	Strong inhibitors of CYP450 3A3/4 may raise ziprasidone levels.

Due to its propensity to cause prolongation of the QTc interval, drug interactions with ziprasidone have been most probed. Ketoconazole (400 mg/day), a potent CYP3A4 inhibitor, administered with ziprasidone (40 mg/day) was found to increase the steady state mean plasma concentrations of ziprasidone by 34%. While the sample size was small ($n = 14$) and only descriptively reported, there appeared to be more adverse events seen with the combination of ziprasidone and ketoconazole (71%) than with ziprasidone and placebo (30%). Dizziness was reported in 36% of those receiving both drugs vs 8% receiving ziprasidone alone. No increases in the QTc interval >500 msec occurred, and no treatment-emergent or significant changes in laboratory measures of vital signs were encountered.

Erythromycin, another commonly used CYP450 specific inhibitor, has not been systematically studied for concomitant use with ziprasidone. Even when employed alone, macrolide antibiotics can prolong QTc intervals by blocking K^+ channels. However, this effect most often occurs with high doses or intravenous administration. However, cases of torsades de pointes have been reported both for erythromycin and clarithromycin when used alone.

Cimetidine is an H_2 receptor antagonist that is known to inhibit several isoforms of CYP450, including CYP3A4. At doses of 800 mg/day, this nonspecific inhibitor increased ziprasidone plasma concentrations by only 6%, an amount that is unlikely to be clinically significant. However, in data presented to the FDA, cimetidine administration did increase the mean baseline QTc by 7.8 msec. In addition to the CYP450 system, approximately 60% of ziprasidone is metabolized by aldehyde oxidase. In contrast to CYP450 enzymes, relatively little is known about the susceptibility of this enzyme to drug, nutritional, and physiologic interactions. Since few medications are metabolized by aldehyde oxidase, the pathway has not been well characterized. However, at least two isoenzymes have been reported to exist. There are some inhibitors and substrates of aldehyde oxidase (Table 13.4). Clinical significance of any of these interactions with ziprasidone has not been studied in humans.

TABLE 13.4 — SUBSTRATES AND INHIBITORS OF ALDEHYDE OXIDASE

Substrate
- Ethanol
- Histamine
- Acetaldehyde

Inhibitor
- Cyclophosphamide
- Pyridoxal (vitamin B_6)
- Menadione (vitamin K_3)
- Dextropropoxyphene
- Methadone
- Diphenhydramine
- Cimetidine
- Chloral hydrate
- Disulfiram

Excretion

The kidney is the major organ for drug excretion. Renal excretion of active drug can be altered by the concurrent administration of any drug that affects renal blood flow, active tubular secretion, or passive tubular reabsorption. These types of interactions with antipsychotics are uncommon. Lithium is one psychotropic that is highly affected by other medications altering these parameters. In the intramuscular (IM) formulation of ziprasidone, the cyclodextrin excipient is cleared by renal filtration. Thus IM ziprasidone should be used with caution in patients with impaired renal function.

13

SUGGESTED READING

Fang J, Gorrod JW. Metabolism, pharmacogenetics, and metabolic drug-drug interactions of antipsychotic drugs. *Cell Mol Neurobiol.* 1999;19:491-510.

Jefferson JW. Drug interactions—friend or foe? *J Clin Psychiatry.* 1998;59(suppl 4):37-47.

Ketter TA, Flockhart DA, Post RM, et al. The emerging role of cytochrome P450 3A in psychopharmacology. *J Clin Psychopharmacol.* 1995;15:387-398.

Maixner SM, Mellow AM, Tandon R. The efficacy, safety, and tolerability of antipsychotics in the elderly. *J Clin Psychiatry.* 1999; 60(suppl 8):29-41.

Shen WW. The metabolism of atypical antipsychotic drugs: an update. *Ann Clin Psychiatry.* 1999;11:145-158.

Tanaka E, Hisawa S. Clinically significant pharmacokinetic drug interactions with psychoactive drugs: antidepressants and antipsychotics and the cytochrome P450 system. *J Clin Pharm Ther.* 1999;24:7-16.

14 Cognition and Antipsychotic Drugs

It is estimated that approximately 40% of patients with schizophrenia have impairments in neuro-cognition. These deficits in cognition are thought to be the result of abnormalities in the frontal and temporal lobes and/or altered connectivity between these regions. The major deficits in patients with schizophrenia are:

- Executive function (abstraction/flexibility)
- Attention
- Verbal fluency
- Learning and memory
- Spatial and verbal working memory
- Semantic memory
- Psychomotor performance.

Functional consequences of these deficits have been found to be clinically relevant. Quality-of-life measures have been highly correlated with cognitive impairment. Executive functioning is related to community functioning, and verbal memory is associated with community function, social problem solving, and skill acquisition. Occupational and social dysfunction are present in most people with schizophrenia. Cognitive deficits prevent many patients with schizophrenia from functioning socially and maintaining employment.

Traditional Antipsychotics

There is no consistent evidence that traditional antipsychotics have positive effects on cognition. Low-potency antipsychotics, such as thioridazine, chlorpromazine, and mesoridazine, may actually worsen working memory, likely due to anticholinergic effects. In fact, cognition has been found to improve in patients once thioridazine is discontinued. Extrapyramidal symptoms (EPS) may also affect motor tasks where speed and accuracy are required. Haloperidol was found to impair higher cognitive functions such as ability to assess one's performance and to shift strategies. Small positive effects have been noted, primarily in attention and semantic memory. Beneficial effects of traditional antipsychotics usually appear only after prolonged treatment and are mainly in sustained attention and visuomotor tasks. Negative effects that occur with acute and chronic treatment with conventional antipsychotics are primarily deficits in attention vigilance and motor skills.

Second-Generation Antipsychotic Drugs

Clozapine has shown some benefits in verbal fluency, semantic memory, attention, and some types of executive functioning. Clozapine has been reported to cause negative results on working memory, possibly due to its dopamine $(D)_1$ antagonist properties, anticholinergic effects, or sedating effects. Risperidone seems to produce different results than those produced by clozapine; patients with schizophrenia who take risperidone have shown improvement in working memory. Risperidone has been shown to improve selective attention, reaction time, alertness, and motor coordination. These effects are possibly due to 5-hydroxytryptamine $(5\text{-HT})_{2A}$ receptor antagonism, the lower rates of EPS, the lower affinity for cholinergic receptors, and the lack of sedation. Treatment with olanzapine has shown improvement in attention, executive functioning, motor skills, learning and memory, and spatial ability. A recent comparative trial found global neurocognitive benefits with risperidone and olanzapine. Risperidone was superior to clozapine and haloperidol for memory improvements. Quetiapine has been associated with improvements in:

- Attention
- Learning
- Verbal reasoning
- Memory
- Executive functioning.

Preliminary data on ziprasidone show improvements in neurocognition similar to those with olanzapine and superior to those with conventional antipsychotics. Improvements were noted for:

- Learning
- Memory
- Attention
- Executive functioning.

Aripiprazole has shown some general improvements in neurocognitive functioning. Verbal memory may be greater with aripiprazole as compared with olanzapine; however, more studies are needed. Although cognitive benefits of these drugs look promising, much work is needed in this area to ascertain the specific cognitive benefits of the second-generation antipsychotic drugs.

Glutaminergic transmission is known to play a fundamental role in cognitive processes. Accumulating evidence suggests that reduced excitatory glutaminergic activity could underlie some symptoms of the disease. Imaging and postmortem studies in patients with schizophrenia have revealed abnormalities in a number of brain regions that are connected by glutamateric circuits. Furthermore, noncompetitive antagonists of N-methyl-D-aspartate (NMDA) receptors, such as phencyclidine and ketamine, exacerbate or produce symptoms and may temporarily decrease cognitive functioning. A family of drugs, the ampakines, enhance

14

excitatory (glutaminergic) transmission and enhance learning and memory in rodents, suggesting this group of drugs may improve cognitive dysfunction in patients. CX516 is in phase II clinical trials and may be promising for improvements in this symptom domain. In a small sample of patients on clozapine, CX516 improved memory and attention on a number of neuropsychiatric tests. This drug may also be beneficial in patients with Alzheimer's disease. Also, cholinesterase inhibitors, such as glantamine and rivastigmine, are undergoing study for improving neurocognition in patients with schizophrenia.

SUGGESTED READING

Collaborative Working Group on Clinical Trial Evaluations. Evaluating the effects of antipsychotics on cognition in schizophrenia. *J Clin Psychiatry*. 1998;59(suppl 12):35-40.

Goldberg TE, Weinberger DR. Effects of neuroleptic medications on the cognition of patients with schizophrenia: a review of recent studies. *J Clin Psychiatry*. 1996;57(suppl 9):62-65.

Green MF, Nuechterlein KH. Should schizophrenia be treated as a neurocognitive disorder? *Schizophr Bull*. 1999;25:309-319.

Jeste DV, Lohr JB, Eastham JH, Rockwell E, Caligiuri MP. Adverse neurobiological effects of long-term use of neuroleptics: human and animal studies. *J Psychiatr Res*. 1998;32:201-214.

Meltzer HY, McGurk SR. The effects of clozapine, risperidone, and olanzapine on cognitive function in schizophrenia. *Schizophr Bull*. 1999;25:233-255.

Rund BR, Borg NE. Cognitive deficits and cognitive training in schizophrenic patients: a review. *Acta Psychiatr Scand*. 1999;100:85-95.

15 Outcomes and Economic Research

Long-term outcomes for many people with schizophrenia remain disappointing. Approximately 10% of people with schizophrenia are at risk for suicide and <20% will be employed in competitive work at any time. Preventing relapse is critical to improving all areas of long-term outcome. Without effective maintenance therapy and with the occurrence of high relapse rates, improving patient functioning and quality of life will not be accomplished.

Relapse and Rehospitalization

Up to one half of all stabilized patients may be readmitted within 1 year following discharge. It is known that the more relapses and periods off medication, the poorer the prognosis and long-term outcome for schizophrenic patients. Medication nonadherence is one of the more significant factors leading to relapse in schizophrenia. In the outpatient setting, nonadherence rates in patients with schizophrenia are as high as 50%. This may be due to:

- Illness-related issues, such as lack of insight
- Treatment-management issues, such as inadequate support
- Drug-related issues, such as intolerable side effects.

Extrapyramidal symptoms (EPS), including dystonic reactions, akathisia, and persistent pseudoparkinsonism, may explain why some patients stop taking antipsychotic medications once discharged from the hospital. Second-generation antipsychotic drugs (SGADs), such as aripiprazole, clozapine, risperidone, olanzapine, and quetiapine, are associated with much better side effect profiles as compared with conventional agents. Thus SGADs theoretically may increase patient adherence due to a better risk-benefit profile with respect to clinical efficacy and adverse effects.

Treatment with conventional antipsychotics has been found to be associated with 1-year recidivism rates around 40% to 50%; however, these rates may be decreased with the combination of depot neuroleptic use and intense therapy. Fluphenazine decanoate in combination with social therapy may lower relapse rates to around 23% per year. Fluphenazine decanoate therapy in combination with intense applied family management was associated with a 26% rehospitalization rate over a 2-year period. Although these results are much improved under optimal conditions, the actual "real-world use" of treatment with therapeutic doses of depot medications is probably associated with a higher rate of recidivism.

There is good evidence that the SGADs are more protective against relapse than are the conventional antipsychotics. One-year rehospitalization rates of treatment-resistant patients receiving clozapine are between 13% and 18% per year. Rehospitalization rates for risperidone, olanzapine, and quetiapine are approximately 12% to 19%. These medications have all been shown to decrease the length of hospital stays as well. Because hospital stays are the primary determinants of overall costs, SGADs can be cost-effective if they are associated with lower rates of rehospitalization.

Quality of Life and Employment

The symptoms and cognitive disturbances of schizophrenia lead to great disability in social and work functioning. Less than 20% of all patients with schizophrenia are employed. In the past, treatment focused on immediate symptom relief, while issues relating to quality of life were largely neglected. Quality of life refers to a patient's subjective sense of well-being. The concept may include:

- Social issues
- Economic well-being
- Fulfillment of personal aspirations
- Relationships.

Other medical or medication issues, such as medication side effects, can relate strongly to the perceived sense of well-being.

The psychiatric field has begun to recognize the importance of these issues in the treatment of schizophrenia. Conventional antipsychotics have produced cognitive and affective impairments influencing well-being, as well as EPS, sexual dysfunction, and tardive dyskinesia, which further lead to a sense of poor quality of life. There is growing evidence that people treated with SGADs compared with conventional agents have a significantly higher general quality of life. This has been reported in long-term treatment with clozapine, olanzapine, risperidone, and quetiapine compared with conventional antipsychotics.

Economics of Schizophrenia

While safety and efficacy of a particular treatment are the primary considerations in selecting an antipsychotic medication, other costs are important to consider as well. The treatment of schizophrenia alone accounts for about 2.5% of the total health care expenditures nationally, with over $32.5 billion being spent in the United States annually. SGADs compared with the conventional agents offer many benefits to treatment, although the higher pricing of SGADs represents a deterrent to their routine use.

Economic analysis techniques are becoming more rigorous and sophisticated as pharmacoeconomic issues are increasingly important in the decision-making process for service providers. There are four principle ways or carrying out economic evaluations as listed in Table 15.1.

TABLE 15.1 — ECONOMIC EVALUATIONS OF SCHIZOPHRENIA	
Analysis Method	**Process**
Cost minimization	This process evaluates the costs of alternative treatment methods. The usual assumption in these studies is that two alternative treatments produce identical outcomes and therefore the least costly method is preferred.
Cost benefit	This analysis compares two treatment approaches and estimates in purely monetary terms the costs and benefits of alternatives. The studies do not include personal costs and benefits since these costs are impossible to evaluate in monetary terms in a realistic way.
Cost-effectiveness	In this analysis, costs are estimated for achieving outcomes such as life-years gained, years of work restored, or time without positive symptoms of schizophrenia.
Cost utility	This analysis requires valid and easily used quality-of-life measures. These results can be combined with survival data to produce estimates of quality-adjusted life-years.

The gold standard for cost-effectiveness analysis is the medical-effectiveness study, a prospective randomized trial designed primarily to obtain cost-effectiveness information. These data can also be obtained by collecting cost data during the typical double-blind, randomized, controlled efficacy trial. Retrospective studies are generally easier to conduct but may be more difficult to interpret. Most published studies involving any of the SGADs and costs are retrospective and/or naturalistic in nature. Although there is little standardization of the variables and methods included in the cost equations, there is consistency in reporting that SGADs are actually more cost-effective or cost-beneficial compared with conventional antipsychotics when total care is measured.

A large prospective comparative trial found clozapine to be superior to haloperidol while costing over $2000 less per patient per year. Several other prospective and retrospective studies found that treatment with clozapine decreased overall costs per patient per year as compared with prior therapy. Pharmacoeconomic research with risperidone has reported a decrease in hospital stays as compared with conventional antipsychotic therapy. Studies have reported an average savings of between $1000 and $5000 per patient per year with risperidone, and similar results have been seen with olanzapine. Little work has been done with quetiapine, and ziprasidone has not yet been marketed. These, too, may prove to be beneficial for cost savings as compared with conventional antipsychotics. There are few data with which to compare the costs among the SGADs. Because all of the drugs appear to decrease the rate of rehospitalization as well as the length of hospital stays, the main differences in costs would be in the use of outpatient services and the drug costs themselves. The cost of risperidone and quetiapine, for the average doses utilized, is approximately one half that of olanzapine and clozapine. A

15

recent comparative study has found lower monthly costs with risperidone—approximately $250 and $560 lower compared with clozapine and olanzapine, respectively. Additional large prospective controlled trials are needed to ascertain specific differences in overall costs among the SGADs.

SUGGESTED READING

Browne S, Garavan J, Gervin M, Roe M, Larkin C, O'Callaghan E. Quality of life in schizophrenia: insight and subjective response to neuroleptics. *J Nerv Ment Dis*. 1998;186:74-78.

Fleischhacker WW, Hummer M. Drug treatment of schizophrenia in the 1990s. Achievements and future possibilities in optimising outcomes. *Drugs*. 1997;53:915-929.

Franz M, Lis S, Pluddemann K, Gallhofer B. Conventional versus atypical neuroleptics: subjective quality of life in schizophrenic patients. *Br J Psychiatry*. 1997;170:422-425.

Lauriello J, Bustillo J, Keith SJ. A critical review of research on psychosocial treatment of schizophrenia. *Biol Psychiatry*. 1999;46:1409-1417.

Lehman AF. Developing an outcomes-oriented approach for the treatment of schizophrenia. *J Clin Psychiatry*. 1999;60(suppl 19):30-35; discussion 36-37.

Lewis M, McCrone P, Frangou S. Service use and costs of treating schizophrenia with atypical antipsychotics. *J Clin Psychiatry*. 2001;62:749-756.

Weiden P, Aquila R, Standard J. Atypical antipsychotic drugs and long-term outcome in schizophrenia. *J Clin Psychiatry*. 1996;57(suppl 11):53-60.

Williams R, Dickson RA. Economics of schizophrenia. *Can J Psychiatry*. 1995;40(suppl 2):S60-S67.

16 Future Directions

We have begun a paradigm shift in the pharmacologic treatment of psychoses. Second-generation antipsychotic drugs (SGADs) are replacing the conventional agents that have been the mainstay of treatment for almost 40 years. While the dopamine theory of psychosis has been tremendously useful in understanding and modeling this disorder, we now know that SGADs may work through other mechanisms of action. Besides being effective for positive and negative symptoms, when compared with conventional agents, SGADs:

- Cause fewer side effects
- Lessen cognitive impairment
- Lead to a better quality of life
- Have antidepressant effects
- Have much lower relapse and rehospitalization rates.

Because of their improved tolerability and outcomes, these drugs hold more promise in patients with affective components and comorbid substance-abuse histories and in young and elderly patients. Thus one important direction for future research would be to better study current SGADs in subpopulations with schizophrenia.

A second important direction for research is to further address and characterize the limitations and differences among the current compounds. Issues such as weight gain, elevated prolactin levels, and the impact on long-term morbidity and mortality should be addressed. The use of antipsychotics in the treatment of acutely agitated or aggressive patients and better

16

characterization of dosing are other important areas for future research.

New formulations of currently marketed compounds may provide increased ease and adherence with use. Risperidone, olanzapine, and ziprasidone are all undergoing study for the depot formulations. Quetiapine is being studied in sachets and slow-release capsules to allow for less-frequent dosing. A fatty acid amide derivative of clozapine is in early development. Implantable pellets for haloperidol and SGADs that could last up to 5 months are also being studied as are combination agents, such as a fluoxetine/olanzapine product.

Several new products are under investigation in phase II and III studies. Zotepine and MDL 100,907 are two agents that were up-and-coming and had differing properties, the inhibition of norepinephrine reuptake and selective 5-hydroxytryptamine $(5\text{-HT})_{2A}$ antagonism, respectively. These two compounds, however, were recently pulled from trials in US markets. Iloperidone (Zomaril) is currently in phase III trials, including a large multinational trial of over 3000 patients. This agent has a high 5-HT–to–dopamine $(D)_2$ affinity and appears to be effective for positive and negative symptoms. It has a receptor-binding profile similar to that of risperidone. The half-life is about 13 to 14 hours and the most common adverse effects are orthostasis, dizziness, and somnolence. DU127090 is nearing phase III trials. This agent is a mixed dopamine agonist/antagonist with 5-HT_{1A} agonist effects. CX516 (Ampalex), which may augment antipsychotics for neurocognition (see Chapter 14, *Cognition and Antipsychotic Drugs*) is in phase II trials, as is PNU 101387 and LU35-138, D_4 antagonists. Preclinical data hint that other emerging compounds may work by other mechanisms such as inhibiting sigma receptors (SR-31742), modifications of glutamate or nicotine, and inhibition of fatty-acid breakdown (SC-111).

As we consider these exciting new medications, we need to keep in mind the continuing limitations of currently marketed drugs and the sparsity of new agents in the next several years. We must be aware that new, effective therapies for schizophrenia will unlikely be simple in their clinical use. As the psychiatric field works to more accurately identify people who are vulnerable to psychosis and to understand brain regions associated with this illness, we should work to more effectively integrate current treatment options with active psychosocial and rehabilitative programming to attempt to provide beneficial treatment for the people we see today. People who suffer from schizophrenia today will benefit from optimized medication therapy. These benefits include marked improvements in functioning and quality of life.

The pharmacotherapy of schizophrenia has evolved from a relatively simple strategy, involving a homogeneous class of medications with a high ratio of behavioral toxicity to beneficial effects to a more complex group of drugs with improved efficacy. There is, however, no magic bullet or correct therapy for all patients. Clinicians should now attempt to optimize therapy for each patient in a highly individualized way.

16

INDEX

Note: Page numbers in *italics* indicate figures;
page numbers followed by t refer to tables.

17

219

17

17

17

17

17

17

17

17

17